OSCEs in Obstetrics and Gynaecology for Medical Students

Iram Hasan, Charlotte Porter-Hope,
Priyanka Shah, Neha Shah

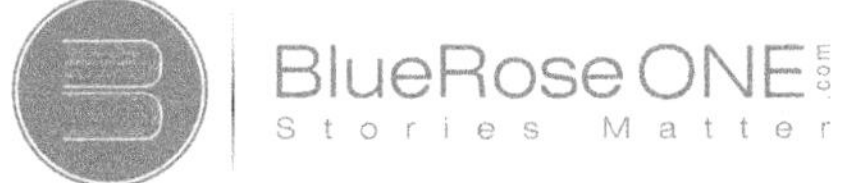

First Published in February 2022

ISBN: 978-93-5427-742-9

BLUEROSE PUBLISHERS

www.bluerosepublishers.com

info@bluerosepublishers.com

+91 8882 898 898

Cover Design:

Aveek

Typographic Design:

Namrata Saini

Preface

An integral part of medical student examinations include OSCEs – Objective Structured Clinical Examinations.

This book aims to make preparing for the Obstetrics and Gynaecology section of the OSCE simpler, by presenting 30 commonly encountered scenarios. Each scenario is presented in a systematic and accessible format including medical student vignettes, patient and examiner briefs with sample mark schemes. Additional information is provided for each scenario to allow for further learning.

Working through these cases will not only make students more prepared for their OSCE examinations but will make them feel more confident in handling common clinical scenarios in their future career.

About the Authors

Iram Hasan MBBS BSc qualified from University College London in 2019 and is currently a Foundation Year Doctor working in Luton. She has a strong interest in Women's Health and hopes to pursue this passion abroad, working in developing countries. She enjoys outdoor sports and learning foreign languages.

Charlotte Porter-Hope MBBS BA qualified from Imperial College London in 2019 and is currently a Foundation Year Doctor working in North London. She enjoys finding new ways to keep fit and experimenting in the kitchen. She is passionate about making medical education accessible throughout her career.

Priyanka Shah MBBS qualified from Brighton and Sussex Medical School in 2019 and is currently a Foundation Year Doctor working in Cambridge. She has received an 'Excellent Teaching Award' from the University of Cambridge and has run regular Obstetrics and Gynaecology teaching sessions. In her spare time, she loves to sing, dance, and bake lots of sweet treats.

Neha Shah MBBS MRCOG qualified from Kings College London in 2012 and is currently an Obstetrics and Gynaecology Doctor working in North London. She is passionate about medical education and has authored several other books within this field. She is currently the Junior Doctor Undergraduate Teaching Lead for Obstetrics and Gynaecology at a North London Hospital.

Contents

OBSTETRICS SCENARIOS:

Antepartum Haemorrhage

Vignette

You are the FY1 on call covering obstetrics. You are bleeped to assess a 28-year-old lady, Amrita Patel, who is 30+4 weeks pregnant and has presented with vaginal bleeding. The midwife is concerned as she is becoming drowsy and less responsive.

Please assess this patient and manage her bleeding.

You have 7 minutes to complete this station.

Patient Brief

You are able to confirm your full name (Amrita Patel) and date of birth (2/4/92). However, you grow tired and are unable to answer further questions.

The midwife then takes over answering the doctor's questions regarding background, further assessment and management.

There is no tenderness on abdominal examination.

Midwife Brief

"My name's Elaine and I'm the midwife covering today. This is Amrita Das, she is 28 years old and 30+4 weeks pregnant. She has come in with heavy vaginal bleeding and I'm worried because she's still bleeding and starting to tire.

I can't find her antenatal notes at the moment, but this is her second pregnancy and she mentioned that she is being followed up for placenta praevia. She previously delivered by Caesarean section 3 years ago.

Her initial observations are: HR 115, BP 92/58, RR 18, T 36.8, SaO2 98% on RA.

The patient has no known drug allergies.

On initial assessment of the bleeding, there is about 500ml on the bedsheet.

There is no tenderness on abdominal examination."

Mark Scheme

<table>
<tr><td>Ensures personal safety</td><td>/1</td></tr>
<tr><td>Washes hands and puts on gloves and gown if available</td><td>/1</td></tr>
<tr><td>Introduces self with full name and role</td><td>/1</td></tr>
<tr><td>Checks for patient response and confirms patient's identity</td><td>/1</td></tr>
<tr><td>Attempts to gain history from patient if responsive, or background from midwife</td><td>/2</td></tr>
<tr><td>Calls for help as patient is drowsy and increasingly unresponsive: senior midwife, obstetrician, anaesthetist, paediatrician, porter and scribe</td><td>/2</td></tr>
<tr><td>Asks for a full set of observations</td><td>/2</td></tr>
<tr><td><u>Airway:</u><ul><li>looks for signs of obstruction such as swelling, secretions or foreign object</li><li>feels for breath</li><li>listens for gurgling, wheezing or stridor</li><li>considers Yankauer sucker for secretions, Magill forceps for visible foreign object, or head tilt-chin lift or jaw thrust if airway obstruction</li><li>positions in left lateral tilt if no airway compromise</li><li>proceeds to assess breathing if patient is talking</li></ul></td><td>/2</td></tr>
<tr><td><u>Breathing:</u><ul><li>looks for cyanosis or signs of difficulty breathing such as use of accessory muscles</li><li>feels for tracheal deviation and symmetrical chest expansion</li><li>percusses chest</li><li>listens to breath sounds (reduced entry, crepitations, wheeze or silent chest)</li><li>asks for respiratory rate and oxygen saturations</li><li>considers an ABG or chest X-ray if desaturating or difficulty breathing</li></ul></td><td>/3</td></tr>
</table>

• gives high flow oxygen (10 to 15l/min) via facemask if oxygen saturations less than 94%	
Circulation: • looks for dry mucous membranes, pallor, active bleeding or other volume losses, and assesses JVP • feels for clamminess, temperature, peripheral oedema and capillary refill time • listens to heart sounds • asks for heart rate, blood pressure, urine output, temperature and an ECG • inserts two large bore cannulas (14G), one in each antecubital fossa • asks for FBC, coagulation screen, U&Es, LFTs, CRP and VBG • considers Kleihauer test if patient is Rhesus D negative • cross matches 4 units of blood • keeps patient warm • checks for any drug allergies • transfuses blood as soon as possible (asks for group specific or O negative blood if there is a delay) • IV fluid resuscitation in the meantime (up to 3.5l: 2l Hartmann's and 1 to 2l colloid) • inserts catheter to monitor urine output	/4
Disability: • assesses pupils' shape, size and reactivity to light • measures glucose • assesses consciousness using AVPU scale or GCS • checks drug chart	/2
Exposure: • fully exposes the patient • palpates the abdomen	/2

<u>Identifies cause of Antepartum Haemorrhage and assesses fetal wellbeing:</u> • performs abdominal and speculum examination • checks last scan for placental location • commences CTG	/3
Continuously reassesses the patient	/1
Behaves in a professional manner	/1
Senior help arrives and candidate provides handover	/2

Additional Information

Definition: Bleeding from the genital tract from 24+0 weeks of pregnancy to before the birth of the baby

- spotting
- minor haemorrhage: less than 50ml and settled
- major haemorrhage: 50 to 1000ml with no signs of clinical shock
- massive haemorrhage: greater than 1000ml and/or signs of clinical shock

Differential diagnoses

- bloody show
- placental abruption
  - part of placenta becomes detached from uterus
- placenta praevia
  - placenta lies in lower uterine segment
- vasa praevia
  - fetus' blood vessels cross or run near the internal os
  - features include ruptured membranes, bleeding and fetal bradycardia
- uterine rupture
  - features shock, pain and bleeding
- abdominal trauma
- cervical polyp
- cervical ectropion
- cervical cancer
- cervicitis
- vaginitis

The most important, although not most common, causes to consider are placenta praevia and placental abruption

Placenta praevia	Placental abruption
• shock proportional to visible loss	• shock disproportional to visible loss
• painless	• constant pain
• soft, non-tender uterus	• tense, tender uterus
• abnormal fetal lie or presentation	• normal fetal lie or presentation

• normal fetal heart	• absent or distressed fetal heart
• small bleeds can lead to larger bleeds	• beware pre-eclampsia, DIC and anuria

Things to note when taking a history and examining

- painful or painless bleeding
    - consider placental abruption if continuous pain
    - consider labour if intermittent pain
- risk factors for placenta praevia or placental abruption
- fetal movements
    - auscultate fetal heart
    - ultrasound if cannot auscultate externally
    - CTG once mother is stable to assess fetal heart rate and aid decision on delivery
- consider ruptured vasa praevia if bleeding is associated with rupture of fetal membranes
- cervical smear history
    - consider neoplastic cervical lesion
- abdominal examination
    - consider placental abruption if tense or woody uterus
    - consider labour if uterine contractions
    - consider placenta praevia, vasa praevia or lower genital tract source if soft and non-tender
- pelvic examination
    - avoid vaginal examinations until placenta praevia excluded
    - speculum to then assess cervical dilatation or lower genital tract cause
    - vaginal examination to assess cervical dilatation if bleeding associated with pain or uterine activity
- ultrasound scan to confirm or exclude placenta praevia if placental site unknown

It is important to document, debrief, handover and carry out clinical incident reporting following these emergencies

Booking appointment

Vignette

You are an F2 on placement at a GP clinic. 23-year-old Rebecca has come in for her booking appointment. Please take a focused history and explain to the mother the antenatal care she will receive during this pregnancy.

Patient brief:

You are a 23-year-old female. You have come in for your booking appointment as you have not had a period for 9 weeks. This is a planned pregnancy which you and your boyfriend are very excited about and you have not experienced any symptoms such as morning sickness.

Obstetric history: You had a medical termination of pregnancy when you were 17 years old. No other pregnancies.

Gynaecological history: Last menstrual period - 9 weeks ago. Your menstrual cycle lasts 29 days and you bleed for 6 days, fairly heavily for which you have used tranexamic acid for 1 year. You were on the Microgynon combined pill from aged 18 until 22. You have not had a smear yet. You last had a sexual health check-up 18 months ago which was negative and since have only had intercourse with your current boyfriend.

Past medical history: You are asthmatic which is well controlled in community with no ITU admissions and is triggered by dust and cold. You have no psychiatric history.

Drug history: You use a Beclomethasone inhaler daily, a Salbutamol inhaler around twice a month and Tranexamic acid for heavy periods. You have no drug allergies.

Family history: You are the youngest of 4 children, which were all vaginal births. Your mother's pregnancies were all uncomplicated and reached full term.

Social history: You smoked 10 cigarettes a day, until 1 year ago; now you occasionally smoke when stressed. You stopped drinking when you discovered you were pregnant 5 weeks ago and used to drink about 4 units a week. You deny recreational drug use. You work as a receptionist at a GP surgery. You live in a flat with your boyfriend of 3 years, David, who is very supportive and caring and who works as a mechanic. There has never been any violence or abuse within the relationship. Your parents live half an hour drive away and are very excited about the pregnancy. You are sure they will be supportive. You have not experienced any low mood recently. You are slightly anxious as this is your first time speaking to a medical professional about your pregnancy.

Mark Scheme

Washes hands	/1
Introduces themself	/1
Determines last menstrual period	/1
Current mood and feelings Determines whether the pregnancy planned	/2
Previous obstetric history	/2
Previous gynaecological history	/2
Past medical history	/2
Drug history	/1
Social history Job and home situation Smoking, alcohol and recreational drug use Asks about safety at home (any abuse or violence) Asks about support from partner and family	/4
Explain which booking bloods and measurements will be done at this appointment. Weight, height, blood pressure, urine dipstick HIV, syphilis, Hepatitis B, blood screening if high risk	/1 /1
Antenatal schedule Explains regular antenatal appointments and purpose Explains which scans will happen and when • Booking and dating scan: 8-14 weeks • Anomaly scan: 18-22 weeks	/4
Explains who the mother should contact if concerns	/1
Antenatal advice Avoid Smoking, alcohol	/1 /1

Certain foods such as unpasteurised milk, raw/undercooked meat/fish/egg Check with clinician before starting new medication Ensures patient taking Folic Acid (until 12 weeks) and Vitamin D (throughout pregnancy)	/1 /1
Caring and understanding patient manner	/3
Total/30	/30

Additional Information

Booking appointments should happen before 10 weeks gestation and serve as an introduction of the mother to antenatal care and pregnancy. This appointment is an opportunity to take a thorough medical and social history to highlight those who may need extra care through the pregnancy including:

- Those with low social support and with experience of domestic violence
- Those who have had female genital mutilation
- Those with any past or present severe mental illness
- Those at risk for gestational diabetes and preeclampsia
- Those with serious medical problems, including cardiac, renal disease, autoimmune conditions, severe asthma and hypertension.

Additionally, the appointment is an opportunity to,

- Check blood group and rhesus D status
- Offer screening for haemoglobinopathies, red cell alloantibodies, anaemia, hepatitis B, HIV and syphilis, asymptomatic bacteriuria
- Discuss and offer trisomy screening (for Downs, Edwards and Patau's syndrome)
- Measure height, weight and calculate BMI
- Measure blood pressure and dip urine for proteinuria

Antenatal care schedule

The antenatal schedule depends on the mother's parity, with those in their first pregnancy having more appointments. Women with medical conditions or risk factors may require additional care. Mothers will receive at least 5 appointments through the pregnancy, to discuss results, check for symptoms, blood pressure and urine dip and to later measure growth of baby and plan the birth.

Additionally, there will be two routine ultrasound appointments

- Dating scan, to determine gestational age, between 11 weeks and 14 weeks.
- Structural anomaly scan, between 18 weeks and 22 weeks.

Pregnancy advice

- Stop alcohol consumption and smoking, refer to cessation services if necessary. Limit caffeine intake.
- Dietary restrictions- avoid raw or undercooked meat, unpasteurized dairy produce, liver and other high vitamin A foods. Limit fish consumption.
- Supplement diet with 10 microgram of Vitamin D per day and 400 micrograms of folic acid per day
- Check with health care professional before stopping or starting medications in pregnancy
- Explain where the mother should turn to for help; for example, may be early pregnancy unit or community midwife team depending on area, urgency and gestation.

CTG Interpretation

Vignette

You are a medical student on the labour ward. Lucy Jones is a 24-year-old lady who is 37+5 weeks pregnant. She has been admitted in early labour for pain control. The team have decided to do a CTG. Once the CTG has been completed, Elaine, a student midwife has a few questions for you.

Please answer her questions and interpret the CTG. You have 10 minutes to complete the station.

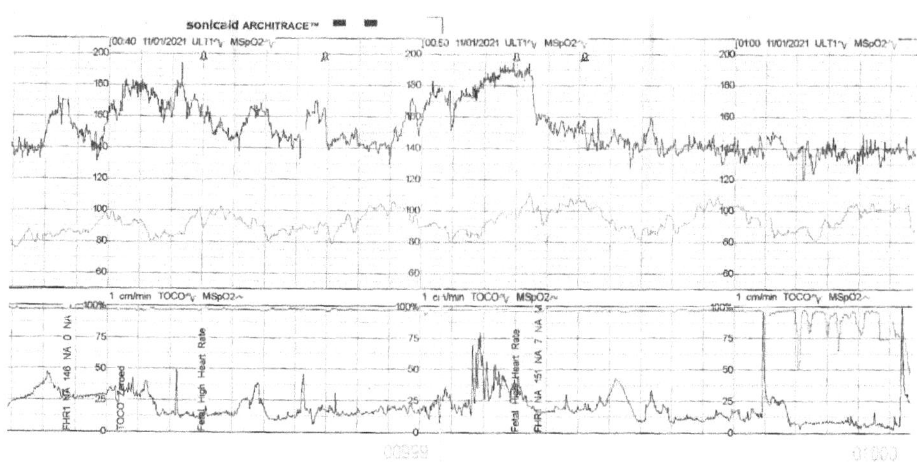

Actor Brief

You introduce yourself and explain that you would like to learn how to interpret a CTG. You find it quite difficult to understand them and you ask if there are any easy ways to learn how to interpret them.

Once you have understood how to interpret a CTG, you then ask what the overall impression is and how should the team manage this patient.

You are also keen to know and ask about:

- Causes of reduced variability
- Different types of decelerations

Mark Scheme

Washes hands	/1
Introduces self with full name and role	/1
Confirms student's identity	/1
Checks students current understanding of the situation and of CTG interpretation	/1
Explains that the CTG is used to monitor the fetal heart and contractions of the uterus.	/1
Explains that it can be used to monitor fetal wellbeing and detect signs of early fetal distress	/1
<u>Define Risk (DR):</u> Identifies that the indication for this CTG is induction of labour. This has been indicated as it has been more than 24 hours since the membranes have ruptured and there are still no contractions.	/2
<u>Contractions (C):</u> Comments that there are 4 contractions in 10 minutes. Comments that intensity can be assessed using palpation.	/2
<u>Baseline Rate (BRA):</u> Comments on an average heart rate of 140 beats per minute in a 10-minute window	/2
<u>Variability (V):</u> Comments on a normal variability between 5 to 25 beats per minute	/2
<u>Accelerations (A):</u> Explains that these are an abrupt increase in baseline fetal heart rate more than 15 beats per minute for more than 15 seconds, and that they are a reassuring feature of fetal wellbeing Correctly comments on the presence of accelerations	/2
<u>Decelerations (D):</u> Explains that these are an abrupt decrease in baseline fetal heart rate more than 15 beats per minute for more than 15 seconds	/2

Comments on the absence of decelerations and that an isolated deceleration is not concerning	
<u>Overall impression (O):</u> Identifies that this is a reassuring CTG as all features are reassuring	/1
Correctly explains that based on the CTG findings, the team will continue CTG monitoring but no further action currently required. Explains that the woman and her birth companion(s) should be updated.	/2
Able to give causes for reduced variability	/2
Able to explain the different types of decelerations and their significance	/3
Behaves in a professional manner	/2
Teaches CTG in bitesize pieces, checking for the student midwives understanding	/2

Additional Information

Define Risk (DR)

- **Maternal illness**: gestational diabetes, hypertension, asthma
- **Obstetric complications**: multiple pregnancy, post-date, previous Caesarean section, intrauterine growth restriction, preterm rupture of membranes, congenital malformations, oxytocin induction, pre-eclampsia
- **Others**: absence of prenatal care, smoking, drug abuse

Contractions (C)

- Aim for 4 contractions in 10 minutes ("4 in 10" or "4:10").

Baseline Rate (BRA)

- **Normal** heart rate: 110-160
- **Fetal tachycardia** more than 160
    - fetal hypoxia, chorioamnionitis, hyperthyroidism, fetal/maternal anaemia, fetal tachyarrhythmia
- **Fetal bradycardia** less than 110
    - post-dates, occiput posterior/transverse presentations

Variability (V)

Fluctuations in baseline heart rate as a result of responses to changes in environment via nervous system, chemoreceptors, baroreceptors and the heart.

- **Normal**: 5-25
- **Reduced variability**:
    - fetus sleeping: normally less than 40 minutes
    - fetal acidosis/hypoxia
    - drugs: opiates, benzodiazepines, methyldopa, magnesium sulphate
    - prematurity: less than 28 weeks
    - congenital heart abnormalities

Accelerations (A)

- Their presence is reassuring especially alongside uterine contractions.
- Their absence with an otherwise normal CTG is of unknown significance.

Decelerations (D)

- **Early**: These are associated with uterine contractions and are due to fetal head compression causing increased vagal tone. They are physiological not pathological.
- **Variable**: These are a rapid fall in baseline heart rate with variable recovery phase. They can be common or seen with umbilical cord compression or oligohydramnios. They are more worrying if persistent or without shouldering.
- **Late**: These begin after the start of a uterine contraction and complete after the end of one. They indicate fetal hypoxia or acidosis as a result of insufficient uterine or placental blood flow. They may be due to maternal hypotension, pre-eclampsia or uterine hyperstimulation. Fetal blood sampling (for pH) or emergency delivery may be required.
- **Prolonged**: These are more than 3 minutes. Causes include uterine rupture, cord prolapse and placental abruption. Consideration should be made for expediting delivery.

Overall Impression (O)

- **Normal:** All features are reassuring
- **Suspicious:** 1 of 3 features is non-reassuring
- **Pathological:** 1 abnormal feature or 2 features are non-reassuring

If the CTG is normal

- continue CTG monitoring
- if it was started because of concerns from intermittent auscultation, remove the CTG after 20 minutes if there are no non-reassuring or abnormal features and no ongoing risk factors.

If the CTG is non-reassuring

- start conservative management
- left lateral position
- oral or IV fluids
- stop oxytocin
- consider tocolysis

If the CTG is abnormal

- offer to take a fetal blood sample or expedite birth after conservative measures

Lactate (mmol/l)	**pH**	**Interpretation**
less than 4.1	more than 7.25	Normal
4.2-4.8	7.21-7.24	Borderline
more than 4.9	less than 7.20	Abnormal

	Baseline (beats/min)	**Baseline variability (beats/min)**	**Decelerations**
Reassuring	110 to 160	5 to 25	None or early Variable with no concerning characteristics for <90 mins
Non-reassuring	100 to 109 161 to 180	<5 for 30 to 50 mins >25 for 15 to 25 mins	Variable with no concerning characteristics for >90 mins Variable with concerning characteristics in <50% of contractions for >30 mins Variable with concerning characteristics in >50% of contractions for <30 mins Late in >50% of contractions for <30 mins with no maternal/fetal clinical risk factors e.g. vaginal bleeding or significant meconium

Abnormal	<100 >180	<5 for >50 mins >25 for >25 mins Sinusoidal	Variable with concerning characteristics in >50% of contractions for 30 mins (less if maternal/ fetal risk factors) Late for 30 mins (less if maternal/fetal risk factors) Acute bradycardia, or single prolonged deceleration >3 mins
NB: Concerning characteristics of variable decelerations include >60s, reduced baseline variability within deceleration, failure to return to baseline, biphasic (W shape), no shouldering NB: If baseline fetal heart rate 100 to 109 with normal baseline variability and no variable/late decelerations, continue usual care			

Category	**Definition**	**Management**
Normal	All features are reassuring	Continue CTG and usual care Update woman and her birth companion(s)
Suspicious	1 non-reassuring feature + 2 reassuring features	Correct underlying causes Full set of maternal observations Start conservative measures Inform obstetrician OR senior midwife Document plan for reviewing CTG and clinical picture Update woman and her birth companion(s) and consider her preferences
Pathological	1 abnormal feature OR	Obstetrician AND senior midwife review Exclude acute events

	2 non-reassuring features	Correct underlying causes Start conservative measures - obstetrician AND senior midwife review if still pathological - offer digital fetal scalp stimulation and document outcome If still pathological following digital fetal scalp stimulation - consider fetal blood sampling - consider expediting birth - consider woman's preferences Update woman and her birth companion(s) and consider her preferences
Need for urgent intervention	Acute bradycardia OR single prolonged deceleration for more than 3 minutes	Urgent obstetric help Expedite birth if acute event - OR acute bradycardia >9 mins (if recovers, reassess) Correct underlying causes Start conservative measures Prepare for urgent birth Update woman and birth companion(s) and consider her preferences
NB: If concerned, consider underlying causes and start conservative measures e.g. encourage mobilisation or alternative position to supine, offer IV fluids if hypotensive, reduce contraction frequency by reducing/stopping oxytocin OR offer tocolytic drug		

Ectopic pregnancy

Vignette

You are clerking in A+E and have been asked to see 28-year-old Suzanne, who is experiencing abdominal pain. Please take the history. Describe the examination and investigations that this patient would need. Explain to the examiner the management options for this patient.

Patient brief

Presenting complaint

You have been experiencing worsening achy suprapubic pain for two days which is not related to position, bowel habit nor improved by analgesia. You noticed a small amount of vaginal dark blood this morning. You have not had any change in bowel habit or urinary symptoms. You took a home pregnancy test last week, as your period was late, which confirmed pregnancy. You are extremely worried you are having a miscarriage and would like to know quickly that the baby is safe.

Gynaecological history

Your last menstrual period was 6 weeks ago. Your periods are normally every 25 days and you bleed for 4 days, not very heavily and restarted postpartum 6 months ago. You have not been using contraception for the past few months as 'you wouldn't mind another child'. You received a course of antibiotics for syphilis when you were 19. Your last STI test was clear, 4 years ago when you first got into a relationship with your fiancée, and he is your only sexual partner currently. Your most recent cervical smear came back positive for HPV, but was not atypical, so you are going back for another smear in a year's time.

Obstetric history

You have one child, who is 14 months old. The pregnancy was uneventful and you had a spontaneous vaginal delivery. You have had no miscarriages or terminations.

Past medical history

You have had no previous surgery. You have hay fever for which you take antihistamines and use eye drops in the spring and summer. You take no regular medication and have no drug allergies.

Social history

You are a police officer. You live with your fiancée and your 14-month child. You have not drunk any alcohol since falling pregnant with your first child as you have been partially breastfeeding since her birth. You do not smoke or take any recreational drugs.

Family history

You have a family history of type two diabetes and coronary heart disease 'in old age'.

On examination

Observations: haemodynamically stable.

Abdominal examination: The abdomen is soft and non-distended with mild suprapubic tenderness.

Pelvic examination: The cervical os is closed, and there is a small amount of dark blood within the vagina. There is some left adnexal tenderness but no masses palpable.

Investigations

Urinary β-hcg: positive

Transvaginal ultrasound scan: Left fallopian tubal pregnancy

Blood tests: pending

Mark scheme

Item	Marks
Introduces self and confirms patient identity	/1
Washes hands	/1
Presenting complaint including last menstrual period	/3
Gynaecological history • Risk factors including previous pelvic infections and surgery • Menstruation and contraception history	 /1 /1
Obstetric history	/2
Other relevant past medical history	/1
Drug history	/1
Social history	/1
Family history	/1
Examination • Basic observations • Abdominal examination • Pelvic examination	/3
Investigations • Urine pregnancy test	/4

• Urine dipstick • Transvaginal ultrasound • Full blood count, C-reactive protein, group and save, serum β-HCG	
<u>Management</u> • Expectant • Medical • Surgical • Dependent on pregnancy size, β-HCG levels, symptoms and patient choice	/7
Carries consultation out with sensitivity	/3
Total	/30

Additional Information

Ectopic pregnancy is the implantation of a fertilised ovum outside of the uterine cavity, most commonly occurring in the fallopian tube. Ectopic pregnancies are non-viable, and they can rupture the structures in which they are implanted in, risking severe haemorrhage. Risk factors for ectopic pregnancy include history of previous ectopic pregnancy, pelvic surgery, pelvic infection, assisted reproduction, being a smoker or using intrauterine contraceptive devices. However, many patients have no identifiable risk factors.

History

Ectopic pregnancy should be suspected in all women of reproductive age presenting with abdominal pain or vaginal bleeding; however some patients may be asymptomatic. Abdominal pain is typically lower pelvic pain, which may be unilateral or generalized, however there is no characteristic character or severity of pain in ectopic pregnancy. There may be accompanying vaginal bleeding. Symptoms are preceded by a period of amenorrhea, typically 5-6 weeks and some women may have already a positive pregnancy test. Ectopic pregnancy symptoms are highly non-specific and it can be clinically difficult to distinguish from early miscarriage. If there is rupture, there may also be gastrointestinal irritation, collapse or dizziness from resulting haemorrhage.

On examination

Haemodynamic stability may be compromised if rupture has occurred. On abdominal examination may demonstrate lower abdominal tenderness, or an acute abdomen, with guarding and rebound tenderness, after rupture. Pelvic examination may be normal in those with an unruptured ectopic pregnancy, but findings can include blood in the vagina, cervical excitation or an adnexal mass or tenderness. If there is an open cervical os, an ongoing miscarriage is likely.

Investigations

All women of reproductive age passing through the emergency department should have a urinary pregnancy test to quickly determine whether there is pregnancy involved. A serum β-HCG level is used to plan management at diagnosis.

If there is a positive urine pregnancy test, transvaginal ultrasound scan is used to locate the pregnancy. In a pregnancy of unknown location, the pregnancy cannot be seen, and repeat serial serum beta HCGs should be offered after 48 hours to determine if the pregnancy is progressing and a further ultrasound is needed.

A patient's full blood count and group and screen should be tested in preparation for potential transfusion, and to determine rhesus status to inform if anti-D is indicated.

Management of tubal ectopic pregnancy

If the patient is unstable, urgent resuscitation is the priority, with administration of blood products if necessary. Tubal ectopic pregnancy can be managed expectantly, medically, or surgically and the choice is based on the risk of rupture and patient choice. Ectopic pregnancies in other locations are assessed and managed differently. Anti-D should be administered to Rh-D negative women who are managed surgically.

Expectant management can be considered if the patient is clinically stable, has well controlled pain and decreasing serum beta-HCG less than 1500iU/L and an unruptured ectopic with adnexal mass smaller than 35mm and no visible heartbeat on ultrasound. Serial β-HCG levels are repeated to ensure consistent decreases, or if further management is indicated. There is a greater likelihood of success in those with lower initial serum β-HCG levels.

Intramuscular methotrexate is used for medical management of ectopic pregnancy. Similarly, to expectant management, eligible women are stable, relatively pain free, with an adnexal mass less than 35mm and can have a serum β-HCG up to 5000 iU/L. Confirmation of absence of a viable intrauterine pregnancy is essential before methotrexate administration. Serial β-HCG measurements are indicated to confirm successful management.

Surgical management is the first line for women who are in severe pain, with signs of a ruptured ectopic, β-HCG greater than 5000 iU/L, or fetal heartbeat or large adnexal mass on ultrasound. It can be also offered as a choice to those who are more stable. If possible, surgery should be laparoscopic, and involves a salpingectomy (removal of whole tube), or salpingotomy (removal of ectopic with tube preservation). Success of surgical management is confirmed with serum β-hcg measurement post salpingotomy and a urinary pregnancy test post salpingectomy.

Gestational Diabetes Mellitus

Vignette

Nina has returned to find out he results of her oral glucose tolerance test at 28 weeks. Take a brief history, explain the following results, the implications for the pregnancy, monitoring and management options.

Fasting blood glucose-5.5

2-hour blood glucose- 8mmol/L

Patient brief

You are a 32-year-old female. You have had no symptoms of diabetes. You were asked to come to screening as you are of South Asian heritage. You have no past medical history and no family history of diabetes. You were normal weight prior to pregnancy. You eat a vegetarian diet which is high in carbohydrates and do not exercise regularly.

This is your first pregnancy which you feel has been going well. You experienced some nausea earlier on but managed to stay well. You are now 28+6 weeks pregnant. You would like a water birth and for it to be 'very natural'.

Ideas, concerns and expectations: You thought diabetes was something 'unhealthy' older people get and didn't realise it could happen in pregnancy. If insulin is mentioned, you are concerned about starting and becoming dependant on it. You are shocked about suggestions to improve diet as have always thought avoiding meat would keep you healthy. You should ask if the problems will go away once the pregnancy is over.

Mark scheme

Introduces themselves and explains reason for consultation	/1
Takes brief history	/2
Checks prior knowledge	/2
Delivers results and explains meaning	/2
Explains gestational diabetes mellitus • Including reference to normal physiology	/2
Avoids use of jargon	/1
Explains implications • Fetus • Mother • Pregnancy	/6
Explains monitoring • Blood glucose monitoring • Extra appointments	/2
Explains management • Lifestyle modifications • Medical management- metformin, insulin • Delivery before 40+6 week gestation, and earlier if on medication/complications	/5
Explains prognosis • Increased risk for future gestational diabetes • Increased risk of future type 2 diabetes, cardiovascular and metabolic disease • Risks are reduced with longstanding lifestyle modifications	/3
Check understanding during and after explanation	/2
Carries out well-structured and clear consultation	/2
Total	/30

Additional Information

During pregnancy, there is progressive insulin resistance, which normally is compensated for by pancreatic β-cell hyperplasia and increased glucose-stimulated insulin secretion. In gestational diabetes mellitus (GDM), there is inadequate pancreatic response, resulting in transient hyperglycaemia. In the majority of cases, there are no symptoms, but can cause polydipsia, polyuria and fatigue.

Complications

GDM and associated hyperglycaemia can result in short and long term implications for mother, infant and pregnancy.

Glucose crosses the placenta, and therefore maternal hyperglycaemia can cause fetal hyperglycaemia and stimulate increased insulin production. These changes induce extra fetal growth, risking development of macrosomia (birth weight greater than 4.5kg) which increases risk of stillbirth and fetal distress. Postnatally, infants are at risk of developing neonatal hypoglycaemia, hyperbilirubinemia, electrolyte abnormalities, polycythemia, respiratory distress and cardiomyopathy. Later in life, offspring have increased risk of developing obesity, impaired glucose tolerance and metabolic syndrome.

During pregnancy, there is an increased risk of maternal gestational hypertension and preeclampsia. If blood sugar is managed with insulin or sulfonylureas, there is a risk of developing hypoglycaemia. Women are at an increased risk of developing type 2 diabetes, cardiovascular disease and metabolic syndrome in the future.

Pregnancies are more likely to be complicated by polyhydramnios. Secondary to macrosomia, there is an increased risk of birth trauma, including brachial plexus injury and fractures, and need for induction of labour, instrumental delivery and caesarean section.

Screening

Screening is offered between 24- and 28-weeks gestation to those with risk factors for developing GDM. These include having a BMI greater than 30 kg/m2, history of delivering a macrosomic baby, first degree family history of diabetes and being from a minority ethnic origin with a high prevalence of diabetes. Mothers with personal history of GDM should be also offered screening shortly after booking as they have a high risk of recurrence.

Oral glucose tolerance tests are used to screen for gestational diabetes. Fasting blood glucose measurements are taken before ingesting 75g of glucose solution. GDM is diagnosed if the fasting blood glucose is greater than 5.6mmol/L or 2 hours post glucose challenge the capillary blood glucose (CBG) is greater than 7.8mmol/L.

Management

Management is introduced in a stepwise and cumulative manner, based on fasting blood glucose at diagnosis, ongoing blood glucose control and evidence of fetal complications, which is shown in figure 1. All women should be advised that lifelong lifestyle changes will improve long term prognosis and overall heath. Glibenclamide can be used as alternative to metformin or insulin therapy if either are declined and monotherapy is insufficient.

Figure 1: Flowchart displaying the addition of management steps in gestational diabetes mellitus.

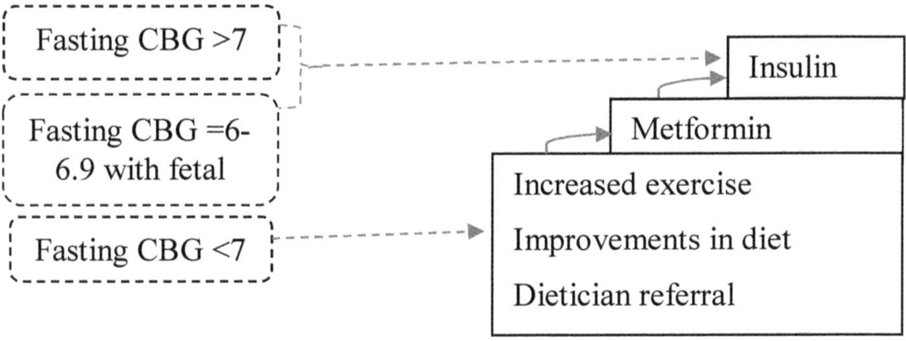

Monitoring requirements

Mothers should record daily fasting and 1 hour post meal blood sugar levels to ensure tight control. Multiple daily insulin regimes require increased CBG monitoring, fasting, pre-meal, 1-hour post meal and at bedtime. Target ranges should be individually tailored however ideally, CBG should be less than 5.3mmol/L when fasting, 7.8mmol/L and 6.4mmol/L one and two hours post meals respectively. If on insulin or glibenclamide, there should be minimum fasting blood glucose set, usually 4mmol/L, to reduce risk of hypoglycaemia.

Timetable

Pregnant women diagnosed with gestational diabetes are seen in joint diabetes and antenatal clinic every 1-2 weeks to monitor blood sugar control. As gestation progresses, the risk of complications increase, and there is additional ultrasound monitoring of fetal growth and amniotic fluid every 4 weeks from 28 to 36 weeks. Women should be advised to deliver before 40 weeks and 6 days and consider earlier induction or caesarean if there is evidence of fetal or maternal complications.

Prognosis

Postnatally, most women will become normoglycaemia as insulin resistance decreases. Women who have had gestational diabetes have a significant risk of developing type 2 diabetes; as GDM reveals borderline pancreatic reserve rather than acting as a causative factor. Women should be offered a fasting plasma glucose test between 6 and 13 weeks postnatally to confirm normoglycaemia; and Hba1c should be monitored annually thereafter. Most women will develop gestational diabetes in later pregnancies. Women will have increased risk of developing metabolic syndrome and cardiovascular disease and should be encouraged to make lifestyle changes to reduce this risk.

Hyperemesis gravidarum

Vignette

You are a final year medical student working on your gynaecology placement. Anjali, a 32-year-old lady, is 10 weeks pregnant and has been referred to the early pregnancy unit due to excessive vomiting. Please take a history, offer relevant examinations and investigations. At 6 minutes, you will receive questions from the examiner.

You have 8 minutes for this station.

Patient brief

Presenting complaint

You are a 32-year-old lady who is 10 weeks pregnant. You visited your GP because your morning sickness has become unbearable. She has referred you to the early pregnancy unit.

History of presenting complaint

You have had morning sickness since the start of pregnancy, but in the last week have been vomiting after everything you eat and barely able to keep water down. You feel very thirsty and dehydrated and your urine seems very concentrated. You were prescribed Cyclizine a few weeks ago but it is no longer helping. There is no blood in the vomit. You feel you are also losing weight, although have not weighed yourself. You sometimes feel dizzy with the dehydration.

You also noticed a small amount of vaginal bleeding yesterday, which you found very concerning. You have not had any other symptoms, including abnormal vaginal bleeding/discharge, abdominal pain, changes to bowels or urine (except going less frequency) or a fever.

Obstetric history

This is your first pregnancy; you have never been pregnant before. During your booking visit, your blood pressure, urine dipstick and all blood tests were unremarkable. You are rhesus negative.

Gynaecological history

Prior to becoming pregnant, you had regular periods on a 31-day cycle. You never passed clots, leaked, or had to use double protection. You had the Mirena coil for contraception but had this removed 3 months ago as you were trying for a baby. Your age of menarche was 13.

Sexual history

You only have sex with your partner, who you have been with for 4 years. You have never been diagnosed with a sexually transmitted infection.

Past medical history

You have no other medical conditions

Past surgical history

Nil

Drug history:

You have been taking 50mg cyclizine three times a day for the vomiting but it is no longer helping. No other regular medications. No known drug allergies.

Family history:

Your mother had breast cancer aged 56; she had a mastectomy and is now under remission. She had no problems during pregnancy. No other family health issues.

Social history:

You live at home with your partner, who is very supportive of your pregnancy. Your parents both live close by. You have never smoked. You used to drink a few beers on the weekends but have not had any alcohol since getting pregnant. Nil recreational drug use.

You work as a sales assistant at a technology company and have had to take the last week off work as you cannot get through the day without vomiting multiple times. You are worried as to why this is happening – you do not really know what is going on but have researched and have heard that having twins can cause excessive vomiting. You are also very concerned about the vaginal bleeding.

On Examination

Clinical signs of dehydration, dry mucous membranes, and increased skin turgor.

Abdominal examination: palpable uterus

Observations: HR 110, BP 100/60, RR 16, O2 saturations 96% on air, Temperature 37.2 degrees

Urine dipstick: ketones +++ nitrites -ve, blood -ve

Weight at booking: 65kg. Weight today: 60kg

Bloods: b-HCG 120,000. AKI stage 1. All other blood tests unremarkable.

Abdominal ultrasound: ‘snowstorm pattern’

Questions at 6 minutes:

1) What is your diagnosis?

Molar pregnancy/Hydatidiform mole

2) Name 3 other risk factors for hyperemesis gravidarum.

Twin pregnancy, raised BMI, first pregnancy

3) What scoring system can be used to classify hyperemesis gravidarum?

Pregnancy-Unique Quantification of Emesis (PUQE) score

4) How would you manage this patient in the immediate scenario, and treat the case?

Immediate: admit to hospital, IV fluids, IV antiemetics, thromboprophylaxis, folic acid and thiamine replacement, consider PPI

Treat the cause: register at a GTD (gestational trophoblastic disease) centre, treat with suction curettage, anti-D prophylaxis. Would need b-HCG monitoring to ensure resolution, with a small chance of needing chemotherapy.

Mark scheme

Introduces themselves, and confirms patients name and date of birth	/1
Establishes how many weeks pregnant the patient is, and asks how the pregnancy has been so far	/1
Takes a history about the vomiting (when started, how many times a day, quantity, content, if anything can be kept down, any haematemesis)	/2
Asks about associated dehydration symptoms (feeling thirsty, dizzy, heart racing, losing weight)	/2
Asks about systemic symptoms (abdominal pain, vaginal bleeding, vaginal discharge, changes to bowel habit, urinary symptoms, fever)	/2
Asks what the patient has already tried to remedy the symptoms	/1
Takes an obstetric history. Establishes that this is a first pregnancy and that booking bloods were normal	/2
Takes a brief gynaecological and sexual history, including menstruation and contraception prior to pregnancy	/1
Asks about past medical history	/1
Asks about past surgical history	/1
Asks about drug history, including over the counter medications and allergies	/1
Asks about family history	/1
Asks about social history (occupation, home situation, smoking and drinking)	/1
Explores the patients, ideas, concerns and expectations	/1
Asks for examination findings – including clinical signs of dehydration and abdominal examination	/1
Asks for relevant investigations – observations, urine dipstick, blood tests (including bHCG), abdominal ultrasound scan	/2
Correctly gives the diagnosis of a molar pregnancy	/1
Correctly names 2-3 other risk factors for hyperemesis gravidarum	/2
Able to name the Pregnancy-Unique Quantification of Emesis (PUQE) score	/1
Offers a reasonable immediate management plan (IV fluids, IV antiemetics, thiamine and folic acid replacement, thromboprophylaxis)	/2

States that the patient will need suction curettage. Will also need anti-D prophylaxis and b-HCG monitoring at a GTD centre to ensure resolution, with chemotherapy needed in resistant cases.	/2
Shows empathy and good patient manner in consultation	/1

Additional Information

Nausea and vomiting in the early stages of pregnancy is not uncommon. It begins in early pregnancy, most commonly between the 4th and 7th week, and usually settles after 12-14 weeks. It is thought to be related to the increasing b-HCG hormone, but it is not clear why it is worse in some women than others. Known risk factors include first pregnancy, multiple pregnancy, previous history of it and molar pregnancy. If this vomiting becomes so severe so as to cause features of dehydration and weight loss, it is called 'hyperemesis gravidarum'.

Hyperemesis gravidarum

This may affect 1-3% of pregnant women. Whilst at home remedies such as eating small amounts and avoiding trigger foods may help, women often need admission to hospital. This is usually the case in the presence of the patient being unable to keep any food/drink down, ketonuria, weight loss and deranged blood tests (AKI/electrolyte abnormalities)

Treatment

Treatment in hospital is usually with IV fluids and IV antiemetics as well as monitoring of observations and urine output. First line antiemetics are antihistamines (H1 receptor antagonists) and phenothiazines (e.g. prochloperazine), although metoclopramide and ondansetron may also be used. Corticosteroids may be needed to refractory cases.

Other considerations

Thiamine can be considered to prevent Wernicke's encephalopathy. Another important consideration for pregnant inpatients is venous thromboembolism prophylaxis, usually with compression stockings and/or prophylactic heparin injections. Remember that pregnant women are at higher risk of VTE.

Gestational trophoblastic disease (GTD)

This is a term that can be used to describe a group of conditions that occur when a pregnancy does not fully develop, with the following two commonest causes:

Partial molar pregnancy:

When two sperm fertilise one ovum, resulting in a fertilised egg with 69 chromosomes (instead of the usual 46). In this case, the fetus may initially seem viable and show signs of development on ultrasound scan – but it cannot survive to term

Complete molar pregnancy:

When an ovum with no chromosomal material (an 'empty' egg) is fertilised by a sperm. The 23 chromosomes from the sperm then divide to produce the normal 46 chromosomes, but it is all paternal. Occasionally two sperm can also fertilise the ovum.

There are also malignant GTD conditions including invasive mole, choriocarcinoma, placental site trophoblastic tumour and epithelioid trophoblastic tumour.

Although GTD is usually suspected on ultrasound, diagnosis is histological.

Risk factors

The main risk factors for developing any of these conditions are:

- Asian origin
- Maternal age <20 or >35
- Previous gestational trophoblastic disease

Symptoms

The commonest symptoms are:

- Vaginal bleeding
- Hyperemesis
- Large for dates uterus

Investigations

An elevated bHCG level may be noted, but diagnosis is usually made by ultrasound scan, showing a characteristic 'snowstorm appearance'. This appears as a central heterogenous mass with multiple cystic areas surrounding it. Note that a partial mole may not have this appearance and is much more difficult to diagnose with ultrasound scan. The differentiation often occurs during histology after treatment.

Treatment

The first line treatment is suction curettage as there is a risk of the trophoblastic tissue remaining in the mother with medical management. However, if the fetus in a partial molar pregnancy is too large, then medical management may be required. All mothers should also be tested for their rhesus status and given anti-D prophylaxis post treatment if they are rhesus negative. Chemotherapy can also be used as an adjunct to all these therapies if bHCG levels do not fall after treatment.

Women diagnosed with gestational trophoblastic disease should be registered at a specialist centre for follow up and to monitor future pregnancies. Standard follow up is at 6 months, during which time contraception is advised.

Hypertension in pregnancy

Vignette

You are a final year medical student working on your obstetrics placement. Maria, a 38-year-old lady, has come in for her 28-week check-up. Please take a history, request any investigations, and offer an appropriate management plan. At 6 minutes, you will receive questions from the examiner.

You have 8 minutes for this station.

Patient brief

History:

You are a 38-year-old lady who has come in for her 28-week check-up. Apart from some difficulty with morning sickness in the early stages, the pregnancy has been uneventful so far. You have just come for a routine check-up and are not experiencing any abnormal symptoms (including headaches, visual disturbances, abdominal pain). You are feeling baby move and kick throughout the day.

During your booking visit, your blood pressure, urine dipstick and all blood tests were unremarkable. Your anomaly scan came back normal and you are rhesus positive.

Obstetric history:

You have one other child who is now 3 years of age. During that pregnancy, you were diagnosed with pregnancy induced hypertension (BP was 150/95) and were treated with oral labetalol. You had weekly blood pressure checks for a few weeks, and the labetalol worked well to control your BP. You were never diagnosed with pre-eclampsia. You went into spontaneous labour at 39 weeks and your daughter was born by vaginal delivery with no complications. You had no issues with hypertension in the post-natal period.

Gynaecological history:

Prior to becoming pregnant, you had regular periods on a 28-day cycle. You occasionally leaked, but rarely passed clots and did not have to use double protection. You were on the combined oral contraceptive pill for 2 years after the birth of your daughter, but since then have not been on any contraception as you were trying to get pregnant. Your age of menarche was 15.

Sexual history:

You only have sex with your husband and have never been diagnosed with a sexually transmitted infection.

Past medical history:

You have a history of hypothyroidism, which is well controlled with levothyroxine.

Past surgical history:

Nil

Drug history:

You take 150 micrograms levothyroxine every morning before breakfast. No known drug allergies.

Family history:

Both your parents have well-controlled hypertension and your mother had pre-eclampsia during her pregnancy.

Social history:

You live at home with your husband, who is very supportive of your pregnancy, and your 3-year-old daughter who is fit and well. You have never smoked. You used to drink a glass of wine on the weekends but have not had any alcohol since trying to get pregnant. Nil recreational drug use. You work as a ward clerk at the hospital, and so would prefer some discretion around your pregnancy. You have lots of friends and family nearby to support you with the pregnancy and feel well prepared as this is your second one. You have not experienced any low mood. You are very excited about having another baby and have no particular concerns.

Examination:

BP: 157/100

Urine dipstick: protein ++, nitrites -ve, blood -ve

SFH: 27cm

All other examinations unremarkable

BMI at booking: 27

Questions at 6 minutes:

1) Name three risk factors for pre-eclampsia.

Previous hypertensive disease in pregnancy, chronic kidney disease, autoimmune disease (such as SLE/antiphospholipid syndrome), type 1 or type 2 diabetes, chronic hypertension, age >40, pregnancy interval of >10 years, BMI >35, family history of pre-eclampsia, multiple pregnancy

2) Name 3 complications of pre-eclampsia.

Eclampsia/seizures, HELLP syndrome, fetal growth restriction, placental abruption, organ damage (acute kidney/liver injury/cardiac failure), long term increase in risk of cardiovascular disease and stroke)

3) How would you manage eclampsia?

Delivery of the baby is the definitive management. Seizures can be treated with IV magnesium sulphate (4g IV bolus, followed by 1g/hour infusion.

Continue treatment until 24 hours after last seizure). Important to monitor urine output, reflexes, respiratory rate and oxygen saturations to avoid Magnesium toxicity.

4) What preventative medication could you offer for high-risk patients?

75-150mg aspirin OD from 12 weeks

Mark scheme

Introduces themselves, and confirms patients name and date of birth	/1
Establishes how many weeks pregnant the patient is, and asks how the pregnancy has been so far	/1
Asks about baby movements	/1
Takes an obstetric history. Establishes previous pregnancy induced hypertension and clarifies how it was managed	/2
Takes a brief gynaecological history, including menstruation and contraception prior to pregnancy	/1
Takes a brief sexual history	/1
Asks about past medical history	/1
Asks about drug history, including allergies	/1
Asks about family history	/1
Asks about social history (occupation, home situation, smoking and drinking)	/1
Explores the patients, ideas, concerns and expectations	/1
Asks for examination findings- specifically BP and urinalysis	/2
Comments on the raised BP and proteinuria to arrive at a diagnosis of pre-eclampsia	/1
Explains the diagnosis of pre-eclampsia to the patient	/1
Assesses for red flag symptoms – headaches, visual disturbance, epigastric pain, oedema	/2
Offers admission and further investigations (FBC, U&Es, LFTs, clotting, urate, urine PCR)	/3
Offers the patient labetalol	/1
Correctly names three risk factors for pre-eclampsia	/2
Correctly names three complications of pre-eclampsia	/2
Offers appropriate management of eclampsia (1- delivery of baby, 1- magnesium sulphate)	/2
Offers aspirin 75-150mg as a preventative measure for high risk pregnancies	/1
Shows empathy and good patient manner in consultation	/1

Additional Information

In normal pregnancy, blood pressure usually falls in the first trimester. Around 20-24 weeks, this then stabilises, and BP will usually increase to pre-pregnancy levels by term. Therefore, any hypertension diagnosed before 20 weeks is categorised as pre-existing. Note that ACE inhibitors and angiotensin receptor blockers have an increased risk of adverse fetal outcomes and so should be changed to an alternative medication during pregnancy.

After 20 weeks, hypertension in pregnancy is defined as:

• systolic > 140 mmHg or diastolic > 90 mmHg

• or an increase above booking readings of > 30 mmHg systolic or > 15 mmHg diastolic

This can then be further categorised into the following:

1) Pregnancy induced hypertension

2) Pre-eclampsia

Pregnancy induced hypertension (PIH), is defined as above, with no proteinuria. It occurs in 5-7% on pregnancies and often resolves after childbirth. It does, however, carry a risk for patients to develop PIH or pre-eclampsia in future pregnancies, as well as hypertension long term.

The difference with pre-eclampsia, is that proteinuria is found on urinalysis. The urine protein: creatinine ratio is used, with a threshold above 30mg/mmol signifying significant proteinuria. It is important to identify as it carries the short-term risks of eclampsia, HELLP syndrome, placental abruption and intrauterine growth restriction. It can also, rarely, develop to multi-organ failure. In long term there is an increased risk of essential hypertension, cardiovascular disease, and stroke.

Risk factors for pre-eclampsia can be divide into high risk and moderate risk:

High risk: hypertensive disease in a previous pregnancy, chronic kidney disease, autoimmune disease, such as systemic lupus erythematosus or antiphospholipid syndrome, type 1 or type 2 diabetes, chronic hypertension

Moderate risk: first pregnancy, age 40 years or older, pregnancy interval of more than 10 years, body mass index (BMI) of 35 kg/m^2 or more at first visit, family history of pre-eclampsia, multiple pregnancy

First line treatment is oral labetalol, or nifedipine if labetalol is contraindicated. BPs above 140/90 should be treated, aiming for a BP <135/85.

High risk groups, or those with two moderate risk factors for pre-eclampsia should 75-150mg once daily aspirin from week 12 of pregnancy until delivery to reduce the chance of developing hypertensive disorders during pregnancy.

Features of severe pre-eclampsia can be noted clinically and through investigations. Patients may complain of headache, blurred vision, epigastric/right upper quadrant pain and peripheral oedema. On examination you may note papilloedema on fundoscopy, hyperreflexia, and abnormal blood test results (low platelets, high creatinine, deranged liver function tests, raised urate).

What is HELLP syndrome?

HELLP stands for **h**aemolysis, **e**levated **l**iver enzymes, **l**ow **p**latelets.

The exact aetiology of why this occurs is unknown, although around 10-20% patients with pre-eclampsia will go on to develop HELLP syndrome. Patient may not be obviously symptomatic, although commonly will present with nausea/vomiting, RUQ pain, and lethargy. The only definitive treatment is delivery of the baby.

What is eclampsia?

Eclampsia is defined as the development of seizures from pre-eclampsia. Magnesium sulphate can be used both to prevent seizures in severe pre-eclampsia, and to treat them. In eclampsia, an IV bolus of 4mg is given, followed by an infusion of 1g/hour until 24 hours after the seizures have stopped. During this time, the patient should be closely monitored, including their urine output, reflexes, respiratory rate, and oxygen saturations. Since magnesium sulphate can cause respiratory depression, it is worth noting that calcium gluconate is the first line treatment for Magnesium toxicity. As with HELLP, the definitive treatment to eclampsia is delivery of the baby.

Labour

Vignette

This is a viva on the stages of labour. Please answer the questions as per the examiner's instructions, giving as much detail as possible.

You have 8 minutes for this station

Examiner's questions

1) Describe what happens in each stage of labour, including definitions of cervical effacement and dilatation

/5

2) Describe the mechanism of labour

/6

3) Describe the possible different lies, presentations and fetal positions

/5

4) Describe the components of the Bishop score and what the score indicates

/6

5) Name 3 ways labour can be induced

/2

6)) What is prelabour rupture of membranes (PROM), how can it be managed and what are the associated complications?

/3

7) What is preterm prelabour rupture of membranes (PPROM), how can it be managed and what are the associated complications?

/3

Mark scheme

Q1) Stage 1 latent phase – painful uterine contractions, including some degree of cervical effacement and dilatation up to 4cm	/1
Stage 1 active phase – painful uterine contractions, a substantial degree of cervical effacement and cervical dilatation from 4cm to fully dilated at 10cm	/1
Stage 2 – from full dilatation to delivery of the fetus	/1
Stage 3 – From delivery of the fetus to when the placenta and membranes have been completely delivered	/1
Cervical effacement involves thinning of the cervix, whereas dilatation involves opening of the cervix	/1
Q2) Engagement – largest diameter of the fetal head descends into the pelvis	/1
Flexion – contractions put pressure on the fetal spine causing the head to flex	/1
Internal rotation – the whole fetus rotates from an occipito-transverse position to occipito-anterior	/1
Extension – the fetal head crowns and there is extension of the presenting part	/1
External rotation/restitution – after the head is delivered, the fetus rotates back to its original position	/1
Delivery of shoulders/rest of body – with the anterior shoulder being delivered first	/1
Q3) Lie: longitudinal, transverse, and oblique	/2
Presentation: cephalic, breech	/1
Position: occipito-anterior (most common), occipito-transverse, occipito-posterior	/2
Q4) See table below: one mark for each correctly described row	/5
A score of < 5 suggests labour is unlikely to start without induction; a score of > 9 suggests labour will likely commence spontaneously	/1
Q5) Membrane sweep, Intravaginal prostaglandins, Oxytocin	/2
Q6) If a pregnant woman's waters break without onset of contractions at 37 weeks of pregnancy or more, there are two options: the first is for immediate induction of labour, or secondly, to wait for labour to start naturally for up to 24 hours. If labour has not commenced within 24 hours, management would usually involve admission, regular observations for signs of chorioamnionitis, intravenous antibiotics and induction of labour.	/3

The main risk is chorioamnionitis.	
Q7) In cases of preterm prelabour rupture of membranes, timing of delivery requires a balance between reducing the risk of prematurity and chorioamnionitis. Patients are usually given intramuscular steroids to reduce the risk of neonatal respiratory distress in the case of preterm labour and commenced on oral antibiotics to reduce the risk of infection. The main risks are prematurity and chorioamnionitis.	/3

Bishop score

	0	1	2	3
Cervical position	Posterior	Intermediate	Anterior	-
Cervical consistency	Firm	Intermediate	Soft	-
Cervical effacement	0-30%	40-50%	60-70%	80+%
Cervical dilatation	<1cm	1-2cm	3-4cm	>5cm
Fetal station	-3	-2	-1,0	+1,+2

Additional Information

The following topics are covered in the mark scheme: stages of labour, mechanism of labour, lies/presentations/fetal positions and the Bishop score. This section will cover further knowledge:

Induction of labour:

There are several indications for inducing labour including: prolonged pregnancy, PROM, maternal diabetes/hypertensive disease, twin pregnancy and suspected in utero fetal compromise.

The main methods of inducing labour are:

Prostaglandins: prostaglandin E2 is thought to cause uterine contraction and softening of the cervix, and can be used in a tablet, gel or pessary form. NICE guidelines currently recommend the use of prostaglandins over oxytocin in women with intact membranes, as they appear to result in greater successful deliveries, and reduced C-section/epidural rates. The primary contraindication for its use is the risk of ovarian hyperstimulation.

Oxytocin: stored in the posterior pituitary gland, oxytocin acts on uterine receptors to cause contractions. It is rarely used alone in patients with intact membranes.

There are also several other options. A membrane sweep can be easily done with an internal examination.

Misoprostol is a drug that is used in termination of pregnancy; currently NICE guidance suggests that it should only be used in induction of labour in cases of intrauterine fetal death.

Finally, there is the option of an amniotomy, or artificial rupture of membrane. This can be effective but often needs augmentation with oxycontin.

Commonly patients will need a combination of these methods, commencing with prostaglandins until it is possible to perform artificial rupture of membranes. After membranes have been ruptures, oxytocin augmentation can be commenced.

Complications of labour:

PROM (prelabour rupture of membranes): this is usually diagnosed through maternal history and speculum exam. If a pregnant woman's waters break without onset of contractions at 37 weeks of pregnancy or more, there are two options: the first is for immediate induction of labour, or secondly, to wait for labour to start naturally for up to 24 hours. If labour has not commenced within 24 hours, management would usually involve admission, regular observations for signs of chorioamnionitis, intravenous antibiotics and induction of labour

Shoulder dystocia: this occurs when the head has been delivered, but the shoulders cannot be delivered with simple traction. It can be associated with perineal tears and haemorrhage in the mother, and brachial plexus injuries in the baby. The primary risk factors and fetal macrosomia, high maternal BMI, and maternal diabetes. It requires urgent assistance.

Placenta praevia: this is commonly known as a low-lying placenta. It is often picked up on the routine 20-week ultrasound scan, with risk factors of multiparity, multiple pregnancy and previous caesarean section. The main symptom is often painless bleeding. Treatment can range from bedrest, to fluid resuscitation, blood product replacement and Caesarean section delivery.

Placental abruption: this is separation of the placenta from the uterine wall, resulting in haemorrhage. Risk factors include pre-eclampsia, multiparity, and maternal age. Symptoms include abdominal pain and vaginal bleeding, and the patient may be in shock which seems out of proportion to their clinical picture. Managed with delivery of the baby and replacement of lost blood products.

Antepartum/postpartum haemorrhage: there are separate stations on these scenarios, but both are clinical emergencies

Uterine rupture: this is a rare but serious complication involving a full thickness tear of the uterine wall. Risk factors can include a previous caesarean section, previous uterine surgery, induction of labour, multiple pregnancy and multiparity. Clinically it can present non-specifically, with sudden severe abdominal pain and/or vaginal bleeding. On examination there can be regression of the presenting part, and there can be clinical features of hypovolaemic shock due to haemorrhage, as well as signs of fetal distress (bradycardia) on CTG. Treatment is with an emergency Caesarean section.

Abnormal lie/presentation/position: Most of these can be diagnosed by ultrasound scan and many will resolve without intervention by the time the baby comes to term. The most common malpresentation that you may come across is a breech presentation, when the baby comes feet or bottom first. Whilst breech babies can be delivered vaginally, a method called 'ECV' (external cephalic version) can be used to turn the baby to a cephalic position. It involves manual manipulation of the fetus to a cephalic presentation through the maternal abdomen and has roughly a 50% success rate. Rare complications can involve rupture of membranes, antepartum haemorrhage and placental abruption. It is not used in women who have had any of these conditions, or in women who have had a previous Caesarean section.

Miscarriage

Vignette

You are an F1 working in an Early Pregnancy Unit where 11-week pregnant Jenny has presented with vaginal bleeding. Please take a focused history and explain what examination and investigations you would like to do. Counsel the patient on the likely diagnosis and her options for management.

Patient brief

Presenting complaint:

Four hours ago, you had a small bright vaginal bleed. This was associated with a slight abdominal 'ache', which 'feels like a period cramp'. You are concerned that you may have hurt the baby when you had sex last night. You have had no infectious contacts recently and have been feeling very well until the abdominal pain and bleeding this morning.

Pregnancy history:

You had mild morning sickness between week 4 and 6 but were able to maintain adequate nutrition. You had your dating scan at 9 weeks, at which the baby 'was healthy and growing well' and 'in the right place'.

Obstetric history:

You have had one previous pregnancy 3 years ago which was delivered at 39 weeks, vaginally, and there were no complications. You have had no previous miscarriages or terminations.

Gynaecological history:

You had a cervical ectropion when started on combined oral contraceptive pill in your early 20s, which caused post coital bleeding at the time. All smears have been normal, and the last one was last year. You have never had any sexually transmitted infections and currently your only sexual partner is your husband.

Past medical history:

You have mild irritable bowel syndrome, which you manage by making changes to your diet.

Drug history:

You take paracetamol for analgesia. You have been taking Folic Acid and Vitamin D supplements as directed by midwife.

Family history:

No family history of clotting disorders or recurrent miscarriage.

Social history:

You live with husband and 2-year-old son, Fred. You are a non-smoker, non-drinker and use no recreational drugs. You are currently not working.

On Examination:

- Observations: Haemodynamically stable

- Abdomen: The abdomen is soft and non-tender
- Pelvic: There is blood draining through cervical os, which is about 3cm open, but no products of conception are visible.

Mark scheme

Introduces themself, confirms patient identity	/1
Washes hands	/1
Introduces themselves	/1
Defined presenting complaint • Characterises bleeding • Characterises pain	/2
Elicits major concerns, ideas and expectations	/2
Obstetric history	/2
Gynaecological history	/2
Past medical history	/2
Family history	/1
Social history	/1
Examination • Observations • Abdominal examination • Vaginal examination; speculum and bimanual examination	/3
Investigations • Ultrasound abdomen and any other appropriate	/2
Explanation • Likely diagnosis of miscarriage • Likely caused by spontaneous genetic abnormality • Management options; expectant, medical and surgical	/7
Carries out history and explanation compassionately and sensitively	/3
Total	/30

Additional Information

A miscarriage is the spontaneous loss of a pregnancy before 24 weeks of gestation. It usually presents with vaginal bleeding and can be accompanied by lower abdominal cramping pain and backache.

Most miscarriages are caused by spontaneous genetic abnormalities in the embryo. Other causes of miscarriage include developmental defects of the placenta or embryo, infection, uterine or cervical abnormality and maternal endocrine or immunological pathologies.

Investigations:

Ultrasonography, usually transvaginal, is used to assess the location and viability of the pregnancy. Viability of pregnancy is based on visualisation of an embryo with cardiac activity. If the fetus or gestational sac are too small to determine if a miscarriage has occurred, a scan is repeated after at least 7 days. If there is lack of growth and continuing absence of cardiac activity, miscarriage can be diagnosed. If the pregnancy location cannot be established, repeat scans and serial serum beta-HCG are necessary to exclude ectopic pregnancy. A laparoscopy is indicated if ectopic pregnancy is considered likely.

Stage of miscarriage:

This is classified based on history, examination, and ultrasound findings.

	Viability	**Symptoms**	**Uterus**
Complete	No	Stopped	Empty
Incomplete	No	Ongoing	Pregnancy tissue remain
Inevitable	No	Ongoing	Pregnancy tissue
Missed	No	None experienced	Empty
Threatened	Yes	Vaginal bleeding	Pregnancy intact

Management:

Missed or incomplete miscarriages should be managed and followed up, to monitor and reduce risk of haemorrhage or intrauterine infection. Choice of management is dependent on clinical state and patient choice.

Expectant management, waiting for pregnancy to terminate without medical or surgical intervention for 7-14 days, is the first line offered for those with incomplete or missed miscarriage. Expectant management is not suitable for those at increased risk of haemorrhage or infection, or with previous adverse pregnancy experiences. If the bleeding and pain settle, a repeat urine pregnancy test is done in 3 weeks and the patient should return to hospital if positive. If the symptoms have not settled or begun within 2 weeks, an ultrasound is repeated, and further options are discussed.

Medical management is offered if expectant management is not appropriate or successful. Vaginal or oral misoprostol stimulates uterine expulsion of products of conception. A repeat pregnancy test is carried out after 3 weeks and women should return if it is positive.

Surgical management is usually offered after expectant or medical management of miscarriage, or for patient choice. Surgical management is either manual vacuum aspiration under local anaesthetic or surgical management under general anaesthetic. Anti-D immunoglobulin should be administered to rhesus-negative women who have receive surgical management of miscarriage.

Pruritus in pregnancy

Vignette

You are clerking in the maternity assessment unit and are asked to review Juliet, a 37-year-old primiparous woman who is complaining of severe pruritus. Please take a history, explain your examination and any appropriate investigations and counsel Juliet on her management options.

Patient brief

Presenting Complaint: You are 34 weeks pregnant and have been experiencing 1 week of intense itch, which started on the palms of your hands and now has spread to most of your body.

History of Presenting Complaint: You have found it very difficult to sleep as the itch is worse overnight and have been struggling to concentrate at work for the last few days. You have experienced no abdominal pain, nausea, headache or fever and you have had no changes in stool or urinary habit. You have had no recent foreign travel and have been in contact with no one who has been unwell recently.

Obstetric history: This is your first pregnancy; it was planned, and you believe it to be 'going smoothly'. You have been experiencing mild back pain for the past 6 weeks. Your baby has been moving well recently. You booked antenatally at 6 weeks and your booking bloods were 'all fine'.

Past Medical history: You had eczema in your childhood and believe this might be a new flare. You experience occasional gastritis, but this has not affected you this pregnancy.

Drug history: You have been taking pregnancy supplements since 6 weeks gestation. You have no drug allergies.

Family history: Your sister experienced itchy skin in her pregnancies, and you remember she had to have multiple blood tests to check 'things were ok'. You have a family history of Parkinson's disease and Prostate cancer.

Social history: You work full time as a carer in a nursing home. You do not smoke and stopped drinking alcohol when you found out you were pregnant, at 6 weeks. You live with your husband who is very supportive and works as an IT technician.

Patient concerns: You are very distressed about the ongoing pruritus and are desperate for medication to stop it immediately. Once informed about the risks to fetus you are very keen to be closely monitored by obstetricians and for regular fetal monitoring.

On examination

Observations: All are stable and within normal limits

Abdominal examination: Non-tender gravid abdomen with symphyseal-fundal height measuring 34cm. There are excoriation marks along all four limbs and across torso and no other skin changes or jaundice.

Investigations (specify only if candidate asks)

Fasting serum bile acids: 45 µmol/L

AST: 200 units/L

ALT: 145 units/L

ALP: 300 units/L

Coagulation: normal

Ultrasound abdomen: no abnormality

Liver screen: negative for alternative hepatic pathology

Mark scheme

<table>
<tr><td>Introduction made and patient identity confirmed</td><td>/1</td></tr>
<tr><td><ul><li>Presenting complaint</li><li>Pruritis history</li><li>Associated symptoms</li></ul></td><td>/2</td></tr>
<tr><td>Pregnancy history</td><td>/2</td></tr>
<tr><td>Past medical history</td><td>/1</td></tr>
<tr><td>Drug history</td><td>/1</td></tr>
<tr><td>Family history</td><td>/1</td></tr>
<tr><td>Social history</td><td>/1</td></tr>
<tr><td>Elicits ideas, concerns and expectations</td><td>/2</td></tr>
<tr><td><u>Examination</u><ul><li>Abdominal examination</li><li>Dermatological examination</li></ul></td><td>/3</td></tr>
<tr><td><u>Investigations</u><ul><li>Aminotransferases and bile acids, clotting profile</li><li>Alternate liver dysfunction causes (including CMV, EBV, autoimmune screen and liver ultrasound)</li></ul></td><td>/3</td></tr>
<tr><td><u>Management options counselling</u><ul><li>Explains slight increased risk to fetus</li><li>Offers symptomatic management and ursodeoxycolic acid</li><li>Offers the choice of intervention after 37 weeks gestation</li></ul></td><td>/5</td></tr>
<tr><td>Carries out consultation sensitively and professionally</td><td>/3</td></tr>
<tr><td>Total</td><td></td></tr>
</table>

Additional Information

Skin changes and pruritus are very common in pregnancy, and pre-existing dermatological conditions are likely to change. The dermatoses of pregnancy are a group of pruritic skin conditions exclusive to pregnancy, described in table 1, note pemphigoid gestationis is diagnosed with skin biopsy and immunofluorescence whereas the remaining two are clinical diagnoses. Obstetric cholestasis is a non-rash forming dermatosis of pregnancy which is described in the following section and excluded from table 1.

Table 1: rash-forming dermatoses of pregnancy

<table>
<tr><th>Dermatosis</th><th>Onset</th><th>Presentation</th><th>Risk to fetus</th><th>Management</th></tr>
<tr><td>Polymorphic eruption of pregnancy</td><td>3rd trimester</td><td>Erythematous papules & urticarial plaques originating in striae gravidarum, sparing umbilicus</td><td>Baby can develop mild rash</td><td rowspan="3">Symptomatic management- emollients, antihistamines, steroids.

(Pemphigoid gestationis may need immunosuppression if severe and non-responsive to steroids)</td></tr>
<tr><td>Pemphigoid gestationis</td><td>2nd trimester onwards</td><td>Urticarial wheals and patches, tense vesicles originate in periumbilical region, striae gravidarum sparing</td><td>Increased risk of prematurity and growth restriction. Baby may develop transient rash</td></tr>
<tr><td>Atopic eruption of pregnancy</td><td>1st trimester</td><td>Dry skin, excoriated erythematous papules or nodules</td><td>nil</td></tr>
</table>

		Face, neck, chest, extensor surface of limbs and trunk		

Obstetric cholestasis

Obstetric cholestasis is characterized by pruritus, in the absence of a rash, with abnormal liver function tests and bile acids, in late second or third trimester of pregnancy. The pathophysiology is not clearly defined but involves poor excretion of bile salts from the liver and increased serum bile salts. The bile salts can cross the placenta and increase the risk of fetal distress, preterm birth and stillbirth, to the greatest extent in mothers with serum bile acid levels greater than 40 µmol/L.

The pruritus of obstetric cholestasis is typically worse at night, widespread and originates in the palms of the hands and the soles of the feet. Secondary skin changes may occur due to excoriation. Abdominal pain, nausea, poor appetite, jaundice and steatorrhea can also occur.

Investigations

Fasting serum bile acid concentrations are elevated in obstetric cholestasis, greater than 11 µmol/L and in severe cases, greater than 40 µmol/L. Serum aminotransferases may also be elevated. In early cholestasis, pruritus can precede biochemical abnormality, and if persistent, transaminases and bile acid levels should be repeated every week. Once obstetric cholestasis is confirmed, liver function tests should be monitored weekly until delivery and return to normal should be confirmed at least ten days postpartum.

Clotting screen should be carried out as can be affected if there is resulting severe liver dysfunction.

Alternative causes of liver dysfunction should be excluded, including screening for viral, autoimmune, and structural causes by blood tests and ultrasound liver.

Management

Women with obstetric cholestasis should be offered symptomatic management of their pruritus, and advised to use cool baths, emollients, and sedating antihistamines to improve quality of sleep.

Ursodeoxycholic acid improves pruritus and liver function but has no effect on fetal outcomes in obstetric cholestasis. Oral vitamin K may be offered if there is clotting dysfunction.

Women with obstetric cholestasis should deliver give birth in a hospital unit under team-based care and should be monitored clinically regularly until delivery.

There is no management available to improve fetal outcomes and it is not currently possible to accurately predict fetal mortality. Mothers should be carefully counselled about the risks and benefits of continuing pregnancy with obstetric cholestasis versus those of induction of labour, to involve in the decision of whether to undergo induction of labour after 37 weeks gestation.

Pruritus normally resolves early in the postpartum period, but there is a high rate of recurrence in subsequent pregnancies.

Obstetric Examination

Candidate Brief

You are a medical student on your obstetrics placement. You have been asked to examine Janet Smith, a 27-year-old lady who is 24 weeks pregnant.

Please perform an obstetrics examination. You have 7 minutes to complete the station.

The examiner will now ask the candidate some questions.

1) What would you do if the symphyseal-fundal height was 20cm?
2) What are the causes of increased fluid (polyhydramnios)?

Mark Scheme

Washes hands	/1
Introduces self with full name and role	/1
Confirms patient's identity	/1
Gains verbal consent and sensitively offers a chaperone	/1
Exposes the patient from below the breasts to the pubic symphysis	/1
Repositions the patient to semi-prone on the bed	/1
Checks for any pain or discomfort	/1
<u>General inspection from the bedside:</u> • appearance • oedema • anaemia • jaundice • pruritic • breathless • weight/height and BMI	/3
<u>Closer inspection of the abdomen:</u> • shape • scars • signs of pregnancy: striae gravidarum, linea nigra, fetal movements (from 24 weeks)	/2
<u>Palpation of the abdomen:</u> • fundus and symphyseal-fundal height • lie • presentation • engagement • fluid: with palpation or percussion	/5

<u>Auscultation of the abdomen:</u> • fetal heart: Doppler US from 12 weeks or Pinard's stethoscope from 24 weeks	/2
Appropriately closes the consultation, thanks the patient and washes hands	/1
Behaves in a professional manner	/1
Summarises findings to the examiner	/3
Appropriately answers question 1: What would you do if the symphyseal-fundal height was 20cm? • Plot this on the patient's Gap-Grow chart (personalised graph for fetal measurements). If this was below the 10th centile, organise an urgent growth scan and follow up	/3
Appropriately answers question 2: What are the causes of increased fluid (polyhydramnios)? • Gestational diabetes, infections (TORCH), fetal abnormalities, idiopathic	/3

Additional information

Shape

- spheroid is reassuring
- ovoid suggests multiple pregnancy, polyhydramnios, transverse lie or fibroids

Scars

- suprapubic suggests lower segment Caesarean section, ectopic pregnancy or ovarian surgery

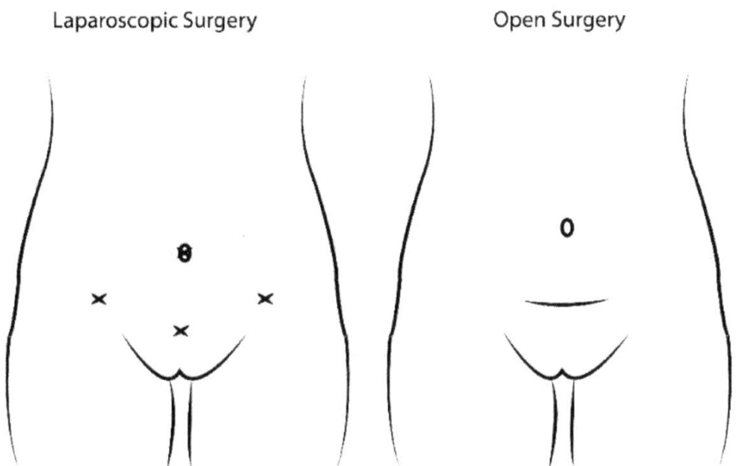

Signs of pregnancy

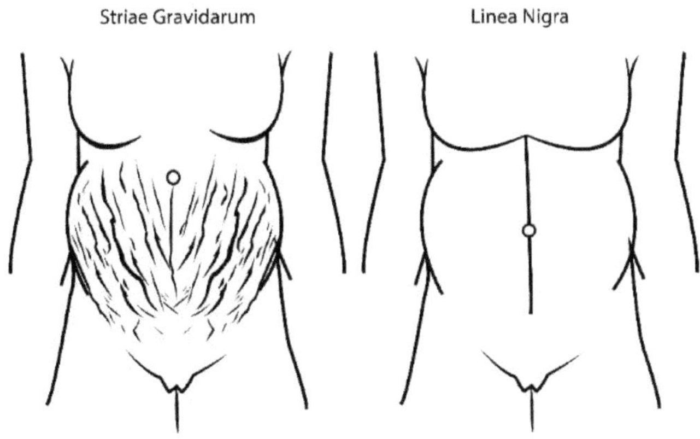

Fundus

- use left hand and measure distance to symphysis pubis

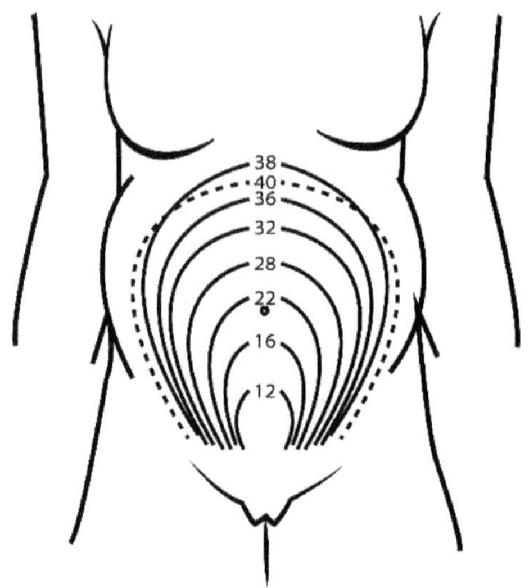

Lie

- relationship of the fetal longitudinal axis to the longitudinal axis of uterus (uterine axis)
- longitudinal, oblique or transverse

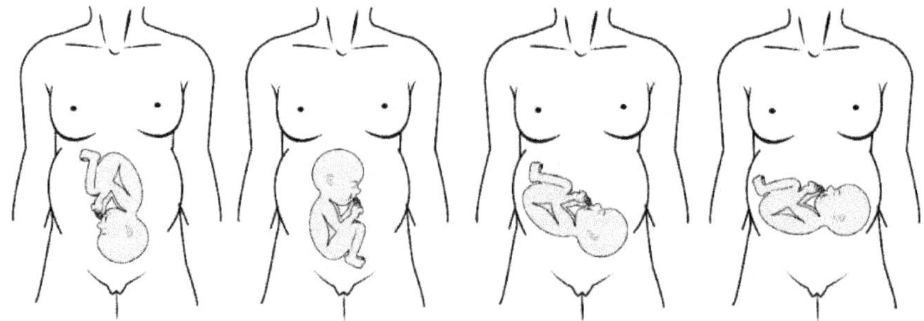

Presentation

- part of fetus overlying the pelvic brim
- hard, round, regular = cephalic
- soft, narrow, irregular = breech

Fetal engagement

- relationship of the fetal head in the pelvis
- less than 2/5 palpable in the abdomen = widest diameter of the presenting part is through the pelvic inlet i.e. the fetal head is engaged

Fluid

- normal
- increased in polyhydramnios, secondary to
    - (gestational) diabetes mellitus
    - fetal abnormality
    - infections (TORCH)
    - idiopathic
    - decreased in oligohydramnios, secondary to
    - pre-term premature rupture of membranes
    - placental insufficiency
    - congenital kidney disease

Auscultation

- auscultate over the anterior shoulder
- shallow groove palpable between the presenting part and rest of fetus
- fetal heart rate should be between 120 and 160 beats per minute

Postnatal Check-up

Vignette

28-year-old Lisa has come in to the GP surgery for a health check 6 week postpartum. Please take a history and explain any examinations and follow up you would like to do.

Patient brief

Pregnancy history:

You experienced no complications during this pregnancy and were well throughout. You, however, experienced a difficult labour, requiring episiotomy and forceps delivery at 41 weeks gestation.

Since birth, you have felt more fatigued, as you have been having difficulty sleeping and getting up throughout the night to feed the baby. You have had painful haemorrhoids and are constipated. You have had no concerns that your perineum is infected or healing poorly after the episiotomy. You have experienced no other new symptoms.

You have not had sex since birth as are concerned about damaging yourself and that it might hurt too much. You would, however, be keen to start contraception as would not like to fall pregnant again soon. You have not had a period since prior to pregnancy.

You have been feeling slightly low, lonely, and isolated from friends and work. You have no thoughts to hurt yourself or baby or any psychotic symptoms.

You have no concerns about your baby's health or growth, and you have been breastfeeding with no problems.

Past obstetric history:

This is your first pregnancy.

Past gynaecological history:

Your periods are normally light, and you bleed for 3 days every 27 days. All of your cervical smears have been normal, you are not due one, and you have never tested positive for any sexually transmitted infections.

Past medical history:

You have a history of eczema, which is controlled well by 'creams'. You have a history of mild depression, which was managed with SSRIs and counselling, and is now resolved.

Drug history:

You have been taking folic acid and iron supplementation since your booking appointment. You are allergic to penicillin (rash).

Social history:

You live with your husband, who you feel well supported by but who works for an international company so works away frequently. You are on maternity leave from your job as a primary school teacher. You are a non-smoker and do not drink alcohol at this time.

Family history:

You have three siblings, and your mother had uncomplicated pregnancies and deliveries for all four children. You have no family history of diabetes or hypertension.

Mark scheme

Introduces self and confirms patient identity	/2
Past medical history	/1
Social history	/1
Family history	/1
Pregnancy history	/2
Delivery history	/2
Maternal postpartum health • Bowel and urinary function • Sexual function • Episiotomy healing • Energy levels • Mental health screening	/7
Screening for domestic violence	/2
Contraception advice and planning	/4
Examination • Weight and blood pressure • Perineal examination	/2
Sensible recommendation for follow up, including postnatal depression screening	/2
Carries out consultation with good patient manner	/4
Total	/30

Additional Information

Postnatal checks are used to review the mother's physical, emotional, and social wellbeing. The postnatal period is also an excellent time to promote healthy lifestyle changes and advice on contraception going forward.

The mother should be counselled regarding regular contraceptives in the postpartum period. At the end of the postnatal period, the coordinating healthcare professional should ensure that the woman's physical, emotional, and social wellbeing is reviewed. Past medical history should also be taken into account.

Conditions specific to pregnancy, such as gestational hypertension, pre-eclampsia, and gestational diabetes, require postnatal follow-up and education regarding the long-term risks and the risk of recurrence in future pregnancies.

Common postpartum complaints:

A comprehensive bodily symptom review is appropriate at postpartum appointments, as pregnancy and labour involve major physiological and anatomical changes. Damage or strain to pelvic floor muscles in pregnancy and childbirth may cause problems with urinary and faecal incontinence and straining in labour can also cause haemorrhoids. Headaches and back pain are also common complaints. Women should be asked about energy levels and, if she was perinatally anaemic, her Full Blood Count should be rechecked. Any vaginal discharge or bleeding should be characterised to ensure there is no signs of infection or prolonged uterine bleeding.

Contraception and intercourse:

Mothers should be asked whether they have resumed sexual intercourse and if they are experiencing dyspareunia or using contraception. Interbirth intervals of at least 2 years are recommended by WHO for both mother and infant health and long-acting methods of contraception should therefore be encouraged. However, if a woman is solely breastfeeding day and night and amenorrheic, there is a low chance of the mother falling pregnant before 6 months.

Mental health and social wellbeing:

At every opportunity postnatally, the mother should be asked about any changes in her mood and mental state to screen for postnatal depression, psychosis, or any other triggered mental health problem. The Edinburgh postnatal depression scale can also be used to detect postnatal depression. Early detection is key in management and minimising the effect on mother and baby. Routinely, questions about the environment and support at home should also be asked, to detect any domestic abuse.

Examination:

A mother's blood pressure and weight should be taken to inform any lifestyle recommendations. If the patient had an episiotomy, perineal tear or caesarean section an examination of the area to assess healing and exclude infection would be appropriate. If the mother mentions problems with urination or passing stool, a vaginal or rectal examination may also be appropriate.

Health promotion and advice:

The postnatal period is a good opportunity to promote a healthy lifestyle. Women who experience gestational hypertension and diabetes are at increased risk of developing these conditions in later life and in future pregnancies and should be advised how to reduce this risk. Any due immunisations should also be advised, and her smear should be rebooked if it was deferred during pregnancy. Weight loss guidance and smoking cessation should be offered if indicated.

A mother should also be asked about breast feeding and guided to appropriate help if she is experiencing any difficulties.

Postnatal depression

Vignette

You are a final year medical student working on your GP placement. Anna, a 24-year-old lady, is three weeks postpartum and has been experiencing low mood. Please take a history, and offer her a management plan. There are no questions in this station.

You have 8 minutes for this station.

Patient brief

Presenting complaint:

You are a 24-year-old lady who had a baby boy three weeks ago and have been experiencing low mood since. Your baby is healthy and growing well but your health visitor noticed your low mood last week and recommended you go to see your GP to discuss this. Your baby is not with you, he is at home with your mother.

History of presenting complaint:

You have been feeling persistently low in mood since you left hospital. You have been struggling to breastfeed and have been using bottled milk, and this makes you feel like you have let your baby down. Because of this, you do not want to spend time with your baby because you feel like you are failing to care for it, and it will eventually be taken away from you. This thought makes you very anxious and you sometimes get palpitations. Your baby is mostly being looked after by your mother and your husband, although he has just gone back to work full time.

You have also been feeling fatigued and have no interest to do anything and have not allowed your friends to visit since giving birth. You cry most days and often struggle to get out of bed. You do not get much sleep during the night when your baby wakes, and when you do fall asleep, you find yourself waking up early. You have not been eating much, despite your mum cooking your meals, and you found you have lost your appetite completely and have lost weight also.

You have been experiencing nightmares of your baby dying, but when awake have not had any visual or auditory hallucinations. You have not had any episodes of mania/elated mood.

You have had thoughts of harming yourself, and sometimes pick at your skin to feel pain, however you have never seriously harmed yourself. You have never had thoughts of harming your baby. You do get suicidal thoughts daily but have never made any plans to go through with it, as you would not want to leave your family behind.

Obstetric history:

You have no other children and have never previously been pregnant. Your baby was born at 36 weeks when you went into spontaneous labour and weighed 3.3kg at birth. You had no complications during pregnancy. As per the health visitor, he has been growing well.

Gynaecological history:

You have not had any cervical smears yet. Prior to pregnancy, you had regular periods, you never leaked, passed clots, or have to use double protection. You have no other gynaecological conditions. Your age of menarche was 11.

Sexual history:

You have been with your current partner for 2 years and have never been diagnosed with a sexually transmitted infection. You have not been sexually active in 6 months and are not on any contraception.

Past medical/psychiatric history:

You have no other medical conditions. You have never suffered from mental health issues in the past.

Drug history:

You do not take any regular medications. You have heard about antidepressants but are worried about trying them because you want to keep trying to breastfeed and do not want anything to get into your breastmilk. You have no known drug allergies.

Family history:

Your sister had puerperal psychosis and nearly took her own life after her baby was born. The child got taken into her father's custody and you are worried the same will happen to you.

Social history:

You live at home with your husband and your new born, although your mum lives close by and visits every day. You have a big support network of friends but have not spoken to any of them/allowed them to visit. Your husband has just gone back to work, and this is making your low mood worse. You have never smoked and gave up alcohol when you found out you were pregnant. You used to smoke cannabis in your teens but nothing recently. You have never experienced domestic violence.

Examination:

All examination findings are unremarkable.

At around 6 minutes, aim to start discussing management options.

Mark scheme

Introduces themselves, and confirms patients name and date of birth	/1
Establishes the reason for coming in and if the patient feels there is any cause for her low mood	/1
Asks about the three core symptoms of depression (low mood, low energy, and low enjoyment)	/2
Establishes if the baby is growing and developing well	/1
Asks about physical symptoms – sleeping and appetite	/1
Asks about symptoms of anxiety - palpitations, breathlessness, sweating	/1
Asks about visual and auditory hallucinations	/1
Asks about episodes of elated mood/mania	/1
Asks about thoughts of self-harm/suicide	/1
Asks about thoughts of harm to the baby	/1
Asks about protective factors that prevent self-harm/harm to baby	/1
Asks about obstetric history – including if any complications during pregnancy/childbirth	/1
Asks about gynaecological/sexual history	/1
Asks about past medical history, specifically psychiatric history	/1
Asks about drug history and allergies	/1
Asks about family history, specifically of mental health issues	/1
Asks about social history (occupation, who is at home and support network)	/1
Asks about smoking, alcohol, and substance abuse	/1
Explores patient's ideas, concerns, and expectations	/1
Offers the chance for the patient to complete the Edinburgh postnatal depression score	/1
Offers a diagnosis of postnatal depression to the patient	/1
Offers a reasonable management plan:	/2

• Conservative – encouraging exercise, support groups, cognitive behaviour therapy, breastfeeding support • Medical – antidepressants, beta blockers, consider thyroid function tests	
Explains that infant exposure to antidepressants through breast milk is extremely low	/1
Explains that antidepressant therapy will not work immediately and may cause mood to worsen before it improves	/1
Offers a leaflet/information about postnatal depression and available support groups	/1
Arranges a follow up appointment in 2-3 weeks	/1
Shows empathy and good patient manner in consultation	/2

Additional Information

The postnatal period can be very emotional, and around 50% of new mothers will experience "baby blues". This can present as tearfulness, irritability and anxiety about the new born, but usually peaks at day 5 postpartum and has usually settled after a couple of weeks without treatment.

However, some women can go onto develop postnatal depression, and in severe cases, puerperal psychosis.

Postnatal depression

This is a mood disorder that occurs after childbirth and can affect both sexes and occurs in 10-15% of women. It can begin during pregnancy or can start several months after childbirth.

Symptoms: Women often experience symptoms very similar to depression including:

- low mood
- irritability
- tiredness and sleeplessness
- change in appetite
- loss of enjoyment
- loss of libido
- negative or guilty thoughts
- anxiety
- thoughts of suicide and self-harm

Risk factors: Although there is no clear cause of postnatal depression, there are several risk factors that increase your likelihood of developing it. These include previous mental health problems (both during and outside of pregnancy), family history of mental health problems, marital difficulties or a poor social support network, a recent stressful event, domestic violence, or previous abuse.

Diagnosis: The Edinburgh postnatal depression score is a tool that can be used alongside history taking in the diagnosis of the condition- it is a short 10 question questionnaire that can help identify postnatal depression, with a score of 10 or more suggesting some level of depression may be present.

Management: Similar to depression outside of pregnancy/childbirth, cognitive behavioural therapy can be used first line. The main issue in that there are often long waiting lists and can be hard to access in some areas. Whilst there is variable evidence on the use of antidepressants, they are often used in clinical practice. It is important to advise patients that they can take 2 weeks to work and often need to be used for at least 6 months to maintain their effects. Most of the older antidepressants have been safely used in breastfeeding for years. St John's Wort is the most commonly used over the counter herbal remedy but advise patients that it can interact with many other medications.

Puerperal psychosis

Puerperal psychosis has an incidence of 1 in 1000 deliveries, and as the name suggests, it can present with manic depression or symptoms of schizophrenia. It also has high suicide rates and can have higher rates of harm to new-borns. Symptoms usually start within the first 2 weeks after childbirth.

Puerperal psychosis needs urgent intervention, and patients or relatives should call their GP, 111, A&E or any known crisis teams. It is usually managed by admission to a special psychiatric unit called a mother and baby unit and medically managed with CBT (cognitive behavioural therapy), antidepressants, antipsychotics, and mood stabilisers. In very severe cases, ECT (electroconvulsive therapy) may be used. The most severe symptoms usually last up to 12 weeks, although it can take up to a year to fully recover.

Postpartum Pyrexia

Candidate Brief

You are the FY1 working on the postnatal ward. You are asked to assess Liliana Evans, a 35-year-old lady, who has had a temperature spike of 38.5 degrees. She gave birth yesterday by Caesarean section and there were no immediate complications. The midwife is concerned as she looks unwell and the patient is becoming increasingly agitated.

Please assess this patient and manage her appropriately.

You have 7 minutes to complete this station.

Patient Brief

You are able to confirm your full name (Liliana Evans) and date of birth (14/6/85) but you become increasingly agitated with further questioning. The candidate is able to calm you down with a good professional bedside manner and you allow them to assess you.

The midwife then takes over answering the doctor's questions regarding background, further assessment and management.

You have abdominal tenderness when examined. There is foul smelling vaginal discharge (lochia) on vaginal examination.

Actor Brief: Midwife

My name's Lizzie and I am the midwife looking after Liliana today. Thank you for coming to see her. I'm a bit worried because she has a fever at the moment, and she generally looks unwell. She is becoming quite agitated too and she seems a little confused. She gave birth yesterday by Caesarean section and there were no immediate complications.

Her initial observations are: HR 100, BP 95/60, RR 18, T 38.5, SaO2 97% on RA.

The patient has no known drug allergies.

The patient has abdominal tenderness when examined. The Caesarean section wound site looks clean and healthy. There is foul smelling vaginal discharge (lochia) on vaginal examination.

The patient improves with the Sepsis Six bundle.

Mark Scheme

Item	Mark
Ensures personal safety	/1
Washes hands and puts on gloves and gown if available	/1
Introduces self with full name and role	/1
Checks for patient response and confirms patient's identity	/1
Attempts to gain history from patient if responsive, or background from midwife	/2
Calls for help as patient is confused and septic	/2
Asks for a full set of observations	/2
Airway: • looks for signs of obstruction such as swelling, secretions or foreign object • feels for breath • listens for gurgling, wheezing or stridor • considers Yankauer sucker for secretions, Magill forceps for visible foreign object, or head tilt-chin lift or jaw thrust if airway obstruction • proceeds to assess breathing if patient is talking	/3
Breathing: • looks for cyanosis or signs of difficulty breathing such as use of accessory muscles • feels for tracheal deviation and symmetrical chest expansion • percusses chest • listens to breath sounds (reduced entry, crepitations, wheeze or silent chest) • asks for respiratory rate and oxygen saturations • considers an ABG or chest X-ray if desaturating or difficulty breathing • gives high flow oxygen (10 to 15l/min) via facemask	/3
Circulation: • looks for dry mucous membranes, pallor, active bleeding or other volume losses, and assesses JVP • feels for clamminess, temperature, peripheral oedema and capillary refill time • listens to heart sounds • asks for heart rate, blood pressure, urine output, temperature and an ECG	/3

• inserts two large bore cannulas (14G), one in each antecubital fossa • asks for FBC, coagulation screen, U&Es, LFTs, CRP, VBG (for glucose and lactate) and blood cultures • checks for any drug allergies • commences IV fluid resuscitation with a STAT 500ml bolus of 0.9% sodium chloride over 15 minutes • starts broad spectrum IV antibiotics such as piperacillin/tazobactam plus clindamycin • inserts catheter to monitor urine output • asks for urine dipstick and sample for culture	
Disability: • assesses pupils' shape, size and reactivity to light • measures glucose • assesses consciousness using AVPU scale or GCS • checks drug chart	/3
Exposure: • fully exposes the patient • examines the breasts • examines the Caesarean section wound for bleeding or oozing • palpates the abdomen • examines the legs for DVT • vaginal examination • takes high vaginal swabs for culture	/3
Continuously reassesses the patient	/1
Behaves in a professional manner	/2
Senior help arrives and candidate hands over	/2

Additional Information

Sepsis is known as the presence of infection combined with systemic manifestations of that infection. Puerperal sepsis can occur from birth to 6 weeks post-partum.

The qSOFA score can be used to quickly identify those with suspected infection, who are at a higher risk of mortality. They must have more than 2 of

- altered mental state
- respiratory rate more than 22 breaths/minute
- systolic blood pressure less than 100mmHg

The most common source of puerperal sepsis is the genital tract resulting in endometritis. Features include

- abdominal or pelvic pain and tenderness
- offensive vaginal discharge
- delay in uterine involution
- heavy lochia

It is important to send high vaginal and placental swabs for culture and to perform pelvic ultrasound as retained placental tissue can be a causative factor.

However, it is important to consider other causes such as

- mastitis or breast abscess
    - examine the breasts
    - send swabs and expressed breast milk for culture
- urinary tract infection
    - urine dipstick
    - send urine sample for culture
- pneumonia
    - chest X-ray
    - send sputum sample for culture
- skin or soft tissue infection
- examine intravenous cannula or injection sites
- examine caesarean or episiotomy wounds
    - send swabs for culture if any discharge
- examine regional anaesthesia site
- gastroenteritis
    - send stool sample for culture including Clostridium difficile
- pharyngitis
    - send throat swab for culture

- bacterial meningitis
    - send CSF for culture
- venous thromboembolism (VTE)
    - pregnancy and the post-partum period can put women at an increased risk of VTE
    - can present with similar features to sepsis
        - increased respiratory rate
        - tachycardia
        - fever
        - crackles on chest auscultation
    - ensure patient is on thromboprophylaxis
    - request compression duplex ultrasound if clinical suspicion of DVT
    - request ECG, chest X-ray and CTPA (or V/Q scan depending on local guidelines) if clinical suspicion of PE

The treatment of sepsis can be easily summarised with the Sepsis Six (give three and take three)

- give high flow oxygen
- give intravenous fluids
- give intravenous antibiotics
- take blood cultures
- take (measure) serum lactate
- take (measure) urine output

It is important to inform the paediatricians so that they can assess and manage the baby appropriately. It is useful to liaise with the microbiologists regarding treatment.

Postpartum Haemorrhage

Candidate Brief

You are the FY2 on call covering obstetrics. You are bleeped to assess a 32-year-old lady, Laura Dowling, who is heavily bleeding following a normal vaginal delivery 20 minutes ago. The midwife is concerned as she is becoming drowsy and less responsive.

Please assess this patient and manage her bleeding.

You have 7 minutes to complete this station.

Patient Brief

You are able to confirm your full name (Laura Dowling) and date of birth (1/2/1988) however you grow tired and are unable to answer further questions.

The midwife then takes over answering the doctor's questions regarding background, further assessment and management.

Midwife Brief

"My name's Tania and I am the midwife covering today. This is Laura Dowling, a 32-year-old who has just delivered 20 minutes ago. It was a normal vaginal delivery, but she is heavily bleeding and becoming unresponsive.

Her initial observations are: HR 120, BP 90/55, RR 16, T 37.1, SaO2 97% on RA.

The patient has no known drug allergies. The patient is not known to have hypertension or pre-eclampsia.

On initial assessment of the bleeding, there is about 1L on bedsheet.

The PPH is from atony and improves if fluid resuscitation, and mechanical and pharmacological management are commenced."

Mark Scheme

Ensures personal safety	/1
Washes hands and puts on gloves and gown if available	/1
Introduces self with full name and role	/1
Checks for patient response and confirms patient's identity	/1
Attempts to gain history from patient if responsive, or background from midwife	/2
Calls for help as patient is drowsy and increasingly unresponsive - senior midwife, obstetrician, anaesthetist, porters and scribe	/2
Asks for a full set of observations	/1
Airway: • looks for signs of obstruction such as swelling, secretions or foreign object • feels for breath • listens for gurgling, wheezing or stridor • considers Yankauer sucker for secretions, Magill forceps for visible foreign object, or head tilt-chin lift or jaw thrust if airway obstruction • proceeds to assess breathing if patient is talking	/3
Breathing: • looks for cyanosis or signs of difficulty breathing such as use of accessory muscles • feels for tracheal deviation and symmetrical chest expansion • percusses chest • listens to breath sounds (reduced entry, crepitations, wheeze or silent chest) • asks for respiratory rate and oxygen saturations • considers an ABG or chest X-ray if desaturating or difficulty breathing • gives high flow oxygen (10 to 15l/min) via facemask regardless of oxygen saturations	/3
Circulation: • looks for dry mucous membranes, pallor, active bleeding or other volume losses, and assesses JVP • feels for clamminess, temperature, peripheral oedema and capillary refill time • listens to heart sounds • asks for heart rate, blood pressure, urine output, temperature and an ECG	/3

• inserts two large bore cannulas (14G), one in each antecubital fossa • asks for FBC, coagulation screen (including fibrinogen), U&Es, LFTs, CRP and VBG • considers Kleihauer test if patient is Rhesus D negative • cross matches 4 to 6 units of blood • keeps patient warm • checks for any drug allergies • transfuses blood as soon as possible (asks for group specific or O negative blood if there is a delay) • fluid resuscitates in the meantime (up to 3.5l: 2l Hartmann's and 1 to 2l colloid) • gives 1g IV tranexamic acid over 10 minutes • inserts catheter to monitor urine output	
Disability: • assesses pupils' shape, size and reactivity to light • measures glucose • assesses consciousness using AVPU scale or GCS • checks drug chart	/3
Exposure: • fully exposes the patient • palpates the abdomen for uterine tone • vaginal examination to look for tear • examines placental products to ensure complete • recognises that uterine atony is the cause of bleeding • performs uterine massage and bimanual compressions to stimulate contractions • gives 5 units of slow IV oxytocin (can be repeated) • gives 0.5mg of slow IV/IM ergometrine (contraindicated in hypertension) • gives 0.25mg IM carboprost at more than 15 minute intervals (maximum of 8 times) • gives 800 micrograms sublingual misoprostol	/5
Continuously reassesses the patient	/1
Behaves in a professional manner	/1
Senior help arrives and candidate begins to handover	/2

Additional Information

Primary PPH

- more than 500ml blood loss from the genital tract within 24 hours of birth
- minor: 500 to 1000ml blood loss
- major: more than 1000ml blood loss

Secondary PPH

- abnormal or excessive bleeding from the genital tract from 24 hours to 12 weeks after birth
- can be secondary to endometritis
- take high vaginal or endocervical swabs
- start antimicrobial therapy e.g. IV gentamicin and IV clindamycin
- can be secondary to retained products of conception or subinvolution of placental implantation site
- examine products passed and do ultrasound scan
- may require surgical evacuation

	Causes	**Management**
TONE **(most common)**	multiple pregnancies previous postpartum haemorrhage failure to progress in 2nd stage of labour general anaesthesia	uterine massage bimanual compressions 5 units slow IV oxytocin (can be repeated) 0.5mg slow IV/IM ergometrine (if no hypertension) 0.25mg IM carboprost (up to 8 times) 800mcg sublingual misoprostol
THROMBIN	pre-eclampsia pre-existing coagulopathies	correction of clotting abnormalities with blood products
TISSUE	retained placenta placenta accreta	ultrasound scan examine products passed remove retained products

TRAUMA	episiotomy perineal laceration	vaginal examination may need suturing

Resuscitation involves replacing blood products and correcting clotting dysfunction

- 4 units RBC (group specific or O negative)
- 4 units FFP if ongoing bleeding
- 1 pool of platelets if ongoing bleeding and platelets less than 75 x 10'9/l
- 2 pools of cryoprecipitate if ongoing bleeding and fibrinogen less than 2g/l

The WHO recommends giving tranexamic acid in all cases of postpartum haemorrhage

- 1g intravenously over 10 minutes
- 2nd dose after 30 minutes or if bleeding restarts within 24 hours
- contraindicated if known venous thromboembolism in pregnancy

Surgical management incudes

- intrauterine balloon tamponade if uterine atony
- haemostatic brace sutures
- stepwise uterine devascularisation
- internal iliac artery ligation
- selective arterial occlusion or embolisation
- hysterectomy

It is important to document, debrief, handover and carry out clinical incident reporting following these emergencies.

Twin pregnancy

Vignette

You are a junior doctor working in gynaecology. Christine, a 35-year-old lady, has presented for her pregnancy dating ultrasound scan. Please take a brief history (4 minutes) and then communicate the findings of her ultrasound scan and answer any questions she may have (4 minutes).

You have 8 minutes for this station.

Patient brief

Presenting complaint:

You are a 35-year-old lady, who is 12 weeks pregnant, and has presented for a routine ultrasound scan.

Obstetric history:

This is your first pregnancy; you have never been pregnant before. So far, your booking visit, your blood pressure, urine dipstick and all blood tests were unremarkable. You have been taking regular folic acid. You conceived this baby using IVF. You have had problems with morning sickness, but this has been settling well with cyclizine. You have not had any other issues during pregnancy.

Gynaecological history:

Prior to becoming pregnant, you had regular periods on a 28-day cycle. You were using the contraceptive patch until 2 years ago, when you started trying to get pregnant. Your age of menarche was 13.

Sexual history:

You only have sex with your husband, who you have been with for 10 years. You have never been diagnosed with a sexually transmitted infection.

Past medical history:

Nil of note

Past surgical history:

You had an appendicectomy when you were 21.

Drug history:

50mg TDS cyclizine for the vomiting.

400mcg OD folic acid.

No other regular medication. No known drug allergies.

Family history:

Nil of note

Social history:

You live at home with your husband, who is very supportive of your pregnancy. Your parents both live close by. You used to smoke 10/day but quit when you started trying for a baby. You do not drink alcohol. Nil recreational drug use.

You work as a manager of a retail company and have not had any issues at work.

Ultrasound scan: (offer this to the candidate at 4 minutes)

Live twin pregnancy, dichorionic, diamniotic (dizygotic)

Allow candidate to explain the results of the scan

Questions to ask the candidate:

1) What does dichorionic, diamniotic mean?
2) What were my risks for having a twin pregnancy?
3) Will I need additional scans and when?
4) What risks are there with twin pregnancy for me and for the babies?
5) When will I deliver, and will I be able to deliver naturally?
6) I have heard about twin-twin transfusion – can you tell me more about it and if it will affect me?

Mark scheme

Introduces themselves, and confirms patients name and date of birth	/1
Establishes how many weeks pregnant the patient is	/1
Asks about how the pregnancy has been so far, including the booking visit	/1
Takes an obstetric history (gravida and parity, mode of previous deliveries and gestation at delivery)	/1
Takes a brief gynaecological history, including menstruation and contraception before pregnancy	/1
Takes a brief sexual history	/1
Takes a past medical/surgical history	/1
Takes a family history	/1
Asks about social history (occupation, home situation, smoking and drinking)	/2
Explains the ultrasound finding of a twin pregnancy	/1
Explains dichorionic, diamniotic correctly: each twin has its own placenta and amniotic sac (1) can either be non-identical twins where two ova are fertilised by two sperm, or identical where one ova is fertilised by a sperm by then splits into two very early on after conception (1)	/2
Identifies 3 risk factors for twin pregnancy (previous twins, family history, old age, multigravida, fertility treatments, ethnicity)	/2
Explains that the patient will have monthly growth scans from 20 weeks onwards	/1
Identifies risk to babies: Prematurity, IUGR	/2
Identifies maternal risks: Anaemia, pre-eclampsia, gestational diabetes, polyhydramnios	/2
Identifies risks during labour: Preterm labour, PPH, malpresentation, cord prolapse	/2
Gives advice on delivery: Delivery usually planned for 37 weeks, although many twin pregnancies will deliver before that. The option	/2

of vaginal delivery or caesarean section depends on which way the twins are lying at that point, and patients choice	
Explains twin-twin transfusion (when both twins share a network of blood vessels and there is unequal blood flow resulting in a donor with reduced growth and a recipient with heart strain). States it does not occur in DCDA twins	/2
Asks if the patient has understood what has been explained to her, and offers an opportunity for further questions	/1
Offers written information/a leaflet to the patient	/1
Shows empathy and good patient manner in consultation	/2

Additional Information

Twin pregnancy occurs in about one in 80 pregnancies. It is usually picked up at the early pregnancy scans (at 12 weeks), however may also be noted if patients present with symptoms of hyperemesis/other exaggerated symptoms of pregnancy. The uterus may also be palpable early in pregnancy or appear large for dates.

Types of twin pregnancy

There are three main types of twin pregnancy:

Dichorionic diamniotic (DCDA) – this occurs when two eggs are fertilised by two sperm, or a fertilised egg splits very early, resulting in each baby having its own placenta and chorion (outer membrane), and having its own amniotic sac. These twins may be identical or non-identical.

Monochorionic diamniotic (MCDA) – if a fertilised egg splits later in development, it may result in an MCDA babies, where they share a placenta and chorion (outer membrane), but they each have their own amniotic sac. These twins will always be identical.

Monochorionic monoamniotic (MCMA) – this is the rarest type of twin pregnancy, and most associated with complications. It occurs when a fertilised egg splits even later than in MCDA twins and as such, they share both a placenta and chorion, and are in the same amniotic sac.

Risks of twin pregnancy

Whilst many women will have healthy twin pregnancies and deliveries without issue, there are several higher risks associated with twin pregnancy.

Risks to mother: anaemia, hypertension/pre-eclampsia, haemorrhage, gestational diabetes

Risks to baby: prematurity, IUGR, twin to twin transfusion syndrome (TTTS)

TTTS is a rare but dangerous complication of monochorionic pregnancies, which can occur when there is unequal blood flow between both babies, resulting in a 'donor' with reduced blood flow and growth restriction, and a 'recipient' with increased blood flow and issues of hypertension and heart strain.

Additional monitoring

Patients are usually cared for by a consultant-led team. MCDA/MCMA twins will have serial growth scans every 2 weeks from 16 weeks, whereas DCDA twins will have growth scans every 4 weeks from 20 weeks. The anomaly scan is unchanged around 20 weeks.

Pregnant women may also be advised to take iron and folic acid throughout pregnancy, and those at high risk of pre-eclampsia, may be advised to take low dose aspirin from 12 weeks onwards.

Labour

It is perfectly possible for twins to be born through a normal vaginal delivery. However, patients commonly go into preterm labour, and if not, usually have labour induced or an elective Caesarean section. This would occur around 37 weeks for DCDA, 36 weeks for MCDA/MCMA and 35 weeks for multiple pregnancy of more than two. Caesarean sections are often recommended if the first twin is in a breech presentation.

GYNAECOLOGY SCENARIOS

Cervical smear

Vignette

You are a junior doctor working in a GP practice. You have been asked to see Miss Smith, a 25-year-old lady who is due to have her first cervical smear. Please take a brief history and consent her for the procedure. You DO NOT have to perform the procedure.

At 5 minutes, you will be asked to explain the findings of her smear to her. At 7 minutes, you will be asked a question from the examiner.

You have 8 minutes for this station.

Patient brief

Presenting complaint:

You are Julie Smith, a 25-year-old lady who has come into her GP after receiving a letter for her first cervical smear test. You have never had any form of internal examination done before and are very nervous. You know the test is for cervical cancer but have no knowledge beyond this.

Past obstetric, gynaecological and sexual history:

You are currently asymptomatic. Your periods are regular and normal. You do not get any post-coital or inter-menstrual bleeding and have not had any pain or discharge. Your age of menarche was 14. You have never been pregnant. You are not currently sexually active. Your last sexual partner was 6 months ago. You did not use protection but have had a chlamydia and gonorrhoea test since then, which were negative. You have never been diagnosed with a sexually transmitted infection. You are not on any regular contraception. This is your first cervical smear.

Past medical history:

No other medical conditions

Past surgical history:

Nil

Drug history:

You take over the counter paracetamol for occasional headaches. No known drug allergies. You never had the HPV vaccine

Family history:

Nil of note

Social history:

You live at home with your mum, dad and elder sister. You work as a cashier at a local grocery store. You have never smoked and drink a glass of wine on weekends. You do not use recreational drugs. You are nervous about this examination as your elder sister found it quite painful.

At 5 minutes, give these results to the candidate:

Mild dyskaryosis with HPV

At 7 minutes, ask the following questions:

How would you manage CIN II/III?

Mark scheme

Introduces themselves, and confirms patients name and date of birth	/1
Washes hands	/1
Briefly asks about past medical history, surgical history, drugs history, family history and social history	/3
Establishes what the patient already knows about the procedure	/1
Explain the purpose of the smear programme is for early detection of cervical cancer and that smears are recommended every 3 years (age 25-50) and then every 5 years (age 50-65)	/2
Explains that there is a possibility of abnormal smears getting missed, or samples coming back as 'inadequate'	/1
Explains that the patient may require further testing if results abnormal, and may need to go to hospital for colposcopy	/1
Explains what will happen during the procedure (small plastic tube/speculum inserted into the vagina using lubricant, to look at the cervix, and then a brush swept around the cervical to obtain a sample)	/2
Explains that the procedure should not be painful, but may be uncomfortable	/1
Advises the patient that she can stop the procedure at any time	/1
Offers a chaperone	/1
Explains what will happen after the procedure – samples will be sent for HPV testing and if positive, for cytology	/1
Offers a patient information leaflet	/1
Asks the patient for consent	/1
Explains the findings of 'mild dyskaryosis with HPV' as: a) Positive for HPV – - a virus that is usually spread via sexual transmission - several types; the main ones cause either genital warts or cervical cancer - around 80% of sexually active women will have a form of HPV at some form in their life	/4

- no treatment is needed, but due to the higher risk of developing cervical cancer, it requires cells to be tested further	
b) Mild dyskaryosis – - mild changes in the appearance of cells that cover the cervix. Also known as CIN I - these do not signify cancer and the majority of cases will not develop into cancer in the future - will often resolve without treatment within 6 months	/3
In view of the above findings, will need to perform colposcopy, which is a specialised procedure to look at the cervix (neck of the womb) using a microscope and liquids applied to the cervix to highlight any abnormal areas.	/2
Offers the chance for the patient to ask any questions	/1
Shows empathy and good patient manner in consultation	/1
How would you manage CIN II/III? -LLETZ (large loop excision of the transformation zone); cryotherapy	/1

Additional Information

Background

Cervical cancer is a cancer often found in the younger population, with a peak incidence in women ages 25-30. Around 80% of cases are squamous cell carcinoma, and around 20% are adenocarcinoma. It can often be asymptomatic and be picked up during routine cervical cancer screening, however it may present with abnormal vaginal bleeding or discharge, or pelvic pain.

HPV and other risk factors

The biggest risk factor for cervical cancer is infection with the HPV virus (particularly serotypes 16,18 and 33), which is usually spread through sexual intercourse. It can be benign and resolve on its own but is the highest risk factor for developing cervical cancer or its pre-cancerous counterparts. As of 2006-2007, an HPV vaccine was released to the mainstream public, aimed at girls between the ages of 9 and 13. Due to this, we may see a difference in the incidence of cervical cancer. Other risk factors for cervical cancer include, the combined oral contraceptive pill, smoking and multiple sexual partners/early first intercourse.

Cervical screening

In 1988, the cervical cancer screening programme was introduced in the United Kingdom. Women are first offered the test aged 25, and this is repeated every 3 years until the age of 50. After this, it is every 5 years, until the age of 65, where the risk of developing cervical cancer becomes lower. Although screening programmes are done different over time and across different countries, currently in the UK, samples are first sent off for HPV testing. Should this come back negative, no further action is required. Should this come back positive, cells are sent for cytology. At this stage there are several possible outcomes:

Negative cytology. Repeat smear in 12 months

Mild dyskaryosis. Routine colposcopy. Conservative treatment likely.

Moderate dyskaryosis. Urgent colposcopy within 2 weeks. Treatment usually recommended

Severe dyskaryosis. Urgent colposcopy within 2 weeks. Treatment always recommended

Inadequate – repeat smear. If 2 inadequate samples, refer for colposcopy

The first line treatment for CIN II and III is a LLETZ procedure (large loop excision of the transformation zone), or cryotherapy.

Contraception counselling

Vignette

You are a final year medical student working on your GP placement. Alisha, a 27-year-old lady, has come in to discuss contraception. Please take a history, including a brief sexual history, and counsel her on her options. Focus on the combined oral contraceptive pill.

You have 8 minutes for this station.

Patient brief

Presenting complaint:

You are a 27-year-old lady who has come in to discuss contraception. 3 months ago, you entered a new relationship with a man, and would like to start on the pill. You have never tried any other method of contraception in the past.

NOTE: Once the candidate has taken the history, make it clear that you want to try the combined oral contraceptive pill for contraception.

History of presenting complaint:

Your new boyfriend has been your only partner in the past 3 months, and you have been using condoms for contraception. You had one episode of unprotected sex 3 weeks ago, for which you took emergency contraception.

You do not get any postcoital or intermenstrual bleeding and have not had any unintentional weight loss or night sweats. Your age of menarche was 12.

You have struggled with acne since your teenage years and would really like to try an option that will improve that. You get the occasional headache but have never suffered from migraines and have never had an aura. You, nor anyone in your family, have ever had a blood clot or breast cancer in the past. You are fit and well and do not have any symptoms of abdominal pain, dyspareunia, dysuria, or abnormal discharge.

Obstetric history:

You had a medical termination of 1 pregnancy when you were 20 at 5 weeks. No other pregnancies.

Gynaecological history:

You have regular periods on a 28-day cycle, which last 5 days and are slightly painful but not too heavy. You never leak, pass clots, or have to use double protection. You have not started having cervical smears yet. Your last menstrual period (LMP) was 3 weeks ago.

Sexual history:

You only have sex with men, and with your current partner have only had vaginal and oral sex. You have never had sex with anyone outside the UK, known HIV positive or men who have sex with men to your knowledge. You have never paid for or been paid for sex, and you have never injected drugs. You have never been diagnosed with a sexually transmitted infection and your last sexual health screen was 3 months ago, which was negative.

Past medical history:

No other medical conditions

Past surgical history:

Appendicectomy 3 years ago (no complications)

Drug history:

You do not take any regular medications. You are allergic to penicillin and get a rash. You occasionally use paracetamol and ibuprofen over the counter for menstrual cramps.

Family history:

Your sister suffers from migraines; however, you have never had this problem.

Social history:

You are at university, in your final year of doing a master's in psychology. You are doing well, although slightly stressed about completing your dissertation. You do not smoke and drink half a bottle of wine on the weekends. You are happy in your new relationship, and your partner is very supportive and caring. You are aware that the pill is user dependent but believe you will be able to take it appropriately. You are not keen for the coil or implant as you do not want to have a procedure. You also want a method of contraception that can be easily reversed should you want to start a family.

Examination:

BP 128/72

BMI 21

Mark scheme

Introduces themselves, and confirms patients name and date of birth	/1
Establishes why the patient wants to start on the COCP	/1
Takes a brief sexual history of the current relationship (regular partner, gender of partner, type of sex, contraception used, unprotected sex and how managed)	/2
Takes a brief general sexual history (partner outside the UK, known HIV positive, men who have sex with men, paying for/being paid for sex)	/1
Takes a menstrual history (LMP, regularity of cycles, length of periods, dysmenorrhoea/menorrhagia)	/1
Asks about red flag symptoms (inter-menstrual bleeding, post coital bleeding, weight loss, night sweats, symptoms of STIs)	/1
Asks about possible contraindications (migraine with aura, thromboembolic disease, breast cancer, smoking)	/2
Asks about obstetric/gynaecological history	/1
Asks about past medical history	/1
Asks about drug history and allergies (including over the counter medication such as St John's Wort)	/1
Asks about family history (especially of breast cancer, and VTE)	/1
Asks about social history (occupation, home situation, smoking and drinking)	/1
Ideas, concerns, and expectations	/1
Asks to take patient's blood pressure and BMI, and offers pregnancy test and STI screen	/2
Offers different options for contraception (POP, COCP, LARCs)	/1
Offers an explanation as to how the COCP works (inhibiting ovulation, thickening cervical mucus and thinning the endometrium	/1
Explains benefits of COCP (non-invasive, 99% effective with proper use, lighter and less painful periods, control timings of periods, help acne, reduced risk of ovarian/endometrial/colon cancer)	/2
Explains disadvantages of COCP (side effects, breakthrough bleeding, no protection from STIs, user dependent)	/2

Explains serious risks and red flags of COCP (thromboembolic disease, breast cancer, cervical cancer)	/1
Explains the protocol for starting the pill and missed pill advice (includes diarrhoea and vomiting)	/2
Explain that the COCP can interfere with other medications, including antibiotics and over the counter medication (e.g. St John's Wort), therefore to always check with a healthcare provider before starting any new medications	/1
Offers written information to the patient	/1
Shows empathy and good patient manner in consultation	/2

Additional Information

Background

The combined oral contraceptive pill was first approved for use in the United States in 1960 and has become a very popular choice for contraception worldwide. There are three main types of COCP available. The commonest is the monophasic pill, which is taken every day for 21 days with a 7 day 'pill-free' week and with equal amounts of hormone in each pill. The phasic pill is taken in the same way but with differing levels of hormone, and the everyday pill has 7 placebo pills instead of a 7-day break.

Mechanism of action

The COCP works by reducing the release of gonadotrophins and as such, their primary method of action is inhibition of follicular development and subsequent ovulation. This happens through both the oestrogen and progesterone component of the pill. The progestogens produce a negative feedback effect on the hypothalamus, suppressing the release of gonadotropin releasing hormone (GnRH) and subsequently luteinising hormone (LH) and follicle stimulating hormone (FSH). The oestrogen produces a negative feedback effect on the anterior pituitary, thus reducing release of follicle stimulating hormone (FSH) and preventing follicular development. The combination of the two results in immature follicles and no LH surge, so ovulation cannot happen.

Further actions include thickening of the cervical mucus, making it difficult for sperm to penetrate the cervix and reach the upper genital tract, and progestogens can also cause a thinning of the endometrial lining, deterring implantation.

Other uses

The COCP can have many uses above contraception. In Polycystic Ovarian Syndrome, the COCP can help counteract the endometrial hyperplasia caused by unopposed oestrogens, reducing the risk of endometrial cancer. Furthermore, it can be extremely beneficial in improving the symptoms of acne and hirsutism by reducing levels of androgens. In endometriosis, the COCP can suppress the growth of extra-uterine tissue (although not eliminate it), lessening its inflammatory effects and the associated dysmenorrhoea.

Risks

As with any medication, the COCP has its risks, and we use the UK medical eligibility criteria (MEC) to determine whether it can be used safely. These are constantly evolving, but look at risk factors such as BMI, smoking status, thromboembolic disease, breast cancer and migraine with aura alongside many others to aid treatment decisions and determine absolute contraindications.

Other options

When discussing contraception with patients, it is always important to offer different options, including the progesterone only pill (POP), transdermal patch and vagina ring. LARCs are also beneficial as they are not user dependent; these include the depot injection, the implant and both hormonal and copper coils. Since the COCP can affect and be affected by many medications, it is always something patients should be aware of and mention to healthcare professionals.

Dyspareunia

Candidate Brief

You are a final year medical student on your GP placement. You have been asked to take a history from Daniela D'Souza, a 25-year-old lady, who has presented with pain during sexual intercourse.

The examiner will stop you at 7 minutes to ask you a few questions.

Patient Brief

Presenting Complaint:
You introduce yourself (Daniela D'Souza, 17/11/95) and explain that you have started experiencing pain during sex for the past 2 weeks.

History of Presenting Complaint:
You have a sharp stabbing pain during penetration and a dull lower abdominal ache following sex.
You have also noticed increased yellow/green vaginal discharge when wiping and you have had some bleeding after sex. You do not have any skin changes nor changes in your period. You do not have any urinary or systemic symptoms. The pain is mostly associated with sex and it is impacting your relationship. You have never had this type of pain before and painkillers are not helping.

Obstetric and Gynaecological History:
You have never been pregnant. Your last menstrual period was 14 days ago. Your periods normally last 7 days and your cycle is 28 days. You recently had your first cervical screening test and you are awaiting the results. Your last STI check was one year ago, and it was normal.

Sexual History:
You last had sex 3 days ago and it was consensual. This was with your regular partner of 2 months who is male and Portuguese. You had oral and vaginal sex. You are currently on the Pill and you do not use condoms. You have had sex with one other person in the month before you met your current partner.

Past Medical and Surgical History:
You do not have any past medical or surgical history.

Drug History and Allergies:
You are only taking the Pill and you have no known drug allergies.

Family History:
You have no family history of any medical conditions.

Social History:
You work as a shop assistant. You have smoked 5 cigarettes a day since you were 21 and you drink a glass of wine on the weekends with your meal.

Ideas, Concerns and Expectations:
You do not know what is causing the pain, but you are worried about the impact on your relationship.

The examiner will now ask the candidate some questions:

1) What are your differential diagnoses?

2) What investigations would you organise?

Mark Scheme

Item	Mark
Introduces self with full name and role	/1
Confirms patient's identity	/1
Asks an open question to begin the consultation	/1
Establishes if it is superficial or deep dyspareunia	/1
Enquires about time of onset and whether before, during or after sexual intercourse	/1
Enquires about type of pain	/1
Enquires about associated symptoms such as: • genital skin changes, itching or soreness • abnormal vaginal discharge: volume, colour, consistency, smell • abnormal vaginal bleeding: post-coital, intermenstrual, menorrhagia, dysmenorrhoea • abdominal or pelvic pain • dysuria • general malaise, fever, weight loss, rashes or joint swellings	/2
Enquires about course of pain (improving, worsening, or fluctuating) and whether intermittent or constant	/1
Enquires about previous episodes	/1
Enquires about relieving or exacerbating factors	/1
Establishes severity of pain and enquires about effect on life	/1
Takes a gynaecological history: • Date of last menstrual period • Duration and frequency of periods • Abnormal vaginal bleeding • Cervical screening history: last checked, results, any treatment required • STI history: last checked, results, any treatment required	/2
Takes an obstetric history: • Any previous or current pregnancies • Any miscarriages or terminations	/2
Takes a sexual history: • Most recent sexual encounter • Sensitively enquires about consent • Establishes whether regular or casual partner	/2

• Enquires about sex and nationality of partner • Enquires about type of sex • Use of contraception • Enquires about partner's STI history • Enquires about any other partners in last 3 months in the same manner	
Enquires about past medical and surgical history: endometriosis or gynaecological cancers	/1
Enquires about drug history and allergies	/1
Enquires about family history: endometriosis or gynaecological cancers	/1
Enquires about social history • Student or employment status • Living arrangements • Smoking, alcohol and use of recreational drugs	/1
Gains patient's ideas, concerns, and expectations	/1
Appropriately closes the consultation and thanks the patient	/1
Behaves in a professional manner	/1
Explains to the examiner what the differential diagnoses are: • Pelvic inflammatory disease • Endometriosis • Vaginal atrophy • UTI • Functional pain	/2
Explains to the examiner what the next steps are • Examination: systemic, abdominal, bimanual and speculum • Investigations: pregnancy test, high vaginal and endocervical swab, urine dipstick, FBC, U&E, CRP and LFT, US pelvis	/3
	/30

Additional Information

The most common causes of Pelvic Inflammatory Disease are

- Chlamydia trachomatis
- Neisseria gonorrhoeae
- Mycoplasma genitalium

Patients may present with

- lower abdominal pain
- fever
- deep dyspareunia
- dysuria
- menstrual irregularities such as post-coital bleeding, intermenstrual bleeding, dysmenorrhoea or menorrhagia
- vaginal discharge

Patients may have cervical excitation or adnexal tenderness on examination. There may also be some contact bleeding.

Complications include

- perihepatitis (Fitz-Hugh Curtis syndrome)
- chronic pelvic pain
- infertility
- ectopic pregnancy
- abscess

Management includes

- rest
- analgesia
- STI testing
- antibiotics
    - single dose of IM ceftriaxone and 14 days of oral doxycycline and metronidazole
    - 14 days of oral ofloxacin and metronidazole
        - avoid if high risk of gonorrhoea
    - 14 days of oral moxifloxacin
        - avoid if high risk of gonorrhoea
        - effective against Mycoplasma genitalium
    - single dose of IM ceftriaxone and 14 days oral azithromycin
- contact tracing
- offer screening to any male partners within 6 months
- offer 1 week of doxycycline to these partners

- advice against unprotected sexual intercourse until treated and followed up
- advice regarding barrier and long-term contraception

Follow-up includes

- review in 72 hours if moderate to severe symptoms
    - consider further investigations, IV antibiotics or surgery if symptoms not improving
- otherwise review in 2 to 4 weeks
    - check compliance and response to antibiotics
    - check for screening and treatment of contacts
    - test of cure if
        - no abstinence
        - persistent symptoms
        - antibiotic resistance
        - poor compliance or tolerance
        - previous test was positive for chlamydia or gonorrhoea

Emergency Contraception

Student Brief

You are an FY2 working in a GP practice. You are asked to see Alisha Ahmed, a 19-year-old student, who is very anxious and upset as she had unprotected sexual intercourse (UPSI) last night. Please take a history, and counsel the patient regarding emergency contraception and further management options.

You have 7 minutes to complete the station.

Emergency Contraception Counselling

Patient Brief

Presenting Complaint:
You are a 19-year-old student (Alisha Ahmed, 3/10/1990) who has just started University. You are very anxious and upset as you had unprotected sexual intercourse last night with a new boyfriend of two weeks. You would like some emergency contraception as you must not get pregnant. You become very tearful at this as your family do not know that you have a boyfriend and are sexually active.

History of Presenting Complaint:
You had unprotected sex last night with your new boyfriend of 2 weeks. You were both drunk at a party but you both wanted it. You had penetrative and oral sex. You burst into tears when asked if you could be pregnant. You say that you do not know but you have not had sex with him before.

Sexual History:
The last time you had sex was when you were 17 with your ex-boyfriend. You normally use condoms and have never used emergency contraception before. You have not had an STI check, and you do not know if he has but you don't have dyspareunia, unusual vaginal discharge, dysuria nor fevers.

Obstetric and Gynaecological History:
You have never been pregnant in the past and you have never had a miscarriage nor termination of pregnancy. Your last menstrual period was 1 week ago. Your cycle lasts 28 days and your periods are 5 days. You have painful heavy bleeding in the first few days however you have never had intermenstrual bleeding.

Past Medical and Surgical History:
You had childhood asthma. You had an appendicectomy in 2012.

Drug History:
You do not take any regular medication and you do not have any allergies.

Family History:
Your father has hypertension and diabetes. Your mother has migraines (with aura).

Social History:

You are studying PPE at university and you live with flatmates. You are a non-smoker, drink on the weekends and have tried marijuana in the past.

Ideas, Concerns and Expectations:
You become tearful when the doctor explains that there is a risk of pregnancy however you are reassured by the options. You are not keen on an intrauterine device and so you choose to take Ella one. You ask for follow up to discuss future contraception options and you agree to take an STI test.

Emergency Contraception Counselling

Mark Scheme

Washes hands	/1
Introduces self with full name and role	/1
Confirms patient's identity	/1
Asks an open question to begin the consultation	/1
Establishes when she had unprotected intercourse	/1
Establishes what type of sexual activity she had	/1
Establishes if in a relationship or casual partner	/1
Sensitively establishes if any concerns about consent	/1
Establishes if any chance she could be pregnant	/1
Gains a brief sexual history: • any regular contraception or past emergency contraception • how many partners in the past and last sexual encounter prior to this • STI history • any dyspareunia, vaginal discharge, dysuria or fevers	/1
Gains a brief obstetric and gynae history: • any previous pregnancies, terminations, or miscarriages • date of last menstrual period • length of periods and length of cycles • any dysmenorrhoea, menorrhagia, or inter-menstrual bleeding	/1
Past medical history: • rules out hypertension, migraine with aura, asthma, stroke or PE/DVT	/1
Past surgical history	/1
Drug history and allergies:	/1

• rules out steroids, anti-TB medication, anti-epileptic drugs, anti-retroviral therapy, antibiotics, contraception, or St John's wort	
Family history: • rules out stroke, PE/DVT, migraine with aura	/1
Social history: • occupation and housing • alcohol, smoking and use of recreational drugs	/1
Gains patient's ideas, concerns, and expectations	/1
Acknowledges that there is a risk of pregnancy and explains - 80 in 1000 could get pregnant with no emergency contraception - 10 in 1000 could get pregnant with Levonelle - 5 in 1000 could get pregnant with Ella One - 1 in 1000 could get pregnant with IUD	/2
Explains options	/2
Explains side effects and caveats	/3
Advises to seek medical attention if period delayed	/1
Offers long term contraception and an STI check	/2
Provides a leaflet	/1
Appropriately closes the consultation and thanks the patient	/1
Behaves in a professional manner	/1

Additional Information

Earliest ovulation can be estimated to be 14 days before the end of the cycle. Sperm can survive approximately 7 days. The egg can survive approximately 24 hours.

Both Levonelle and Ella One are effective only if taken before ovulation as their primary method of action of delaying ovulation.

	Levonelle (Progestogen)	**EllaOne (Ulipristal acetate)**	**Copper IUD**
Indication	Up to 72 hours after UPSI, and prior to ovulation	Up to 120 hours after UPSI, and prior to ovulation	Up to 120 hours after UPSI or earliest likely ovulation
Effectiveness	95% if less than 24hrs 85% if 24 to 48hrs 58% if 48 to 72hrs Up to 120hrs after UPSI if others contraindicated	More than 98%	More than 99%
Contraindications	Pregnancy Porphyria Reduced effectiveness if BMI over 25, over 70kg or on enzyme inducers (can double the dose)	Pregnancy PPIs, ranitidine, enzyme inducers Severe asthma on oral steroids Hormonal contraception in last 5 to 7 days	Pregnancy Pelvic infection less than 3 months ago (consider oral antibiotics if unsure)
Side effects	Vaginal bleeding	Dysmenorrhoea Pelvic pain	Pain on insertion

	Breast pain Nausea and vomiting Dizziness Headache Diarrhoea	Back pain Nausea and vomiting Headache Dizziness Fatigue Myalgia	Infection risk in 1st 20 days Menorrhagia Irregular bleeding Uterine perforation (2 in 1000 cases) Expulsion (most common in 1st 3 months)
Extra info	Seek medical advice and do a pregnancy test if next period is 5 to 7 days late		
	- Can be used more than once - Seek medical attention if severe lower abdominal pain (small risk of ectopic pregnancy) - Can start hormonal contraception immediately - If vomits within 3 hours, repeat dose with anti-emetic	- Avoid using EllaOne more than once (but FSRH says can be done) - If breastfeeding, express and discard for 7 days - Wait 5 days before starting hormonal contraception - If vomits within 3 hours, repeat dose with anti-emetic	- Return for follow up in 3 to 6 weeks after insertion (if for removal, come in 1st few days after onset of menstruation and must have no UPSI 7 days prior) - Can be removed at any time

Endometriosis

Vignette

You are an FY2 working in general practice. 24-year-old Lavender has made an appointment to discuss her pelvic pain. Take a history, describe examinations and any investigations you would like to do. Counsel Lavender on management options for her symptoms.

Patient brief

Presenting complaint:
You have experienced severe crampy dysmenorrhea for 5 years, occurring throughout your menstrual period, which prevents you from attending work and leaving the house on occasion. You also experience deep dyspareunia, which you have experienced since becoming sexually active 3 years ago, which makes you feel anxious during intercourse. Around your period you also experience pain whilst passing stool (dyschezia) but pass no blood.

Gynaecological history:
Your menstrual cycle lasts for 30 days and you bleed subjectively lightly for 4 days. Your last menstrual period started 10 days ago. Your first menstrual period was at age 13. You use condoms for contraception. You last had a sexual health check 2 months ago which was negative.

Obstetric history:
You have had no previous pregnancies. Although you are not interested in falling pregnant at the present time, you would like to have children when you are older and are concerned about your fertility being affected by this problem. You should specifically ask about if there is anything that can be done to give you the best chances of falling pregnant.

Past medical history:
You have no existing medical problems

Drug history:
You take co-codamol for the pelvic pain, but this does not completely control it. You take no other medications regularly and have no drug allergies

Family history:
Your Mother always had very painful periods but never received any diagnosis or treatment for it. Your father has heart disease and had a myocardial infarction last year. Hayfever runs in your family.

Social history:
You are working as a health care assistant at the local hospital. You live with your boyfriend. You rarely go out when you are experiencing pelvic pain and feel like this means it is more difficult to make new friends at times. You smoke 5 cigarettes a day and drink 10 units of alcohol on the weekends.

Examination:
Pelvic examination: fixed retroverted uterus, no palpable nodules
Abdominal examination: generalized tenderness, no masses palpable

Mark scheme

Introduction and confirmation of patient details	/1
Presenting complaint • Pain • Dyschezia • Dyspareunia • Effect on quality of life	/9
Gynaecological history	/2
Obstetric history	/2
Past medical history	/1
Social history	/2
Family history	/1
Drug history	/1
Examination • Pelvic and abdominal examination	/2
Investigations • Transvaginal ultrasound • MRI, diagnostic laparoscopy or hysterosalpingography may be considered	/2
Management • Medical • Surgical • Fertility treatment	/4
Referral to specialist services offered	/1
Professional and sensitive patient manner	/2
Total	/30

Additional Information

Endometriosis is characterised by endometrial tissue occurring outside of uterus, inducing a chronic inflammatory reaction and the formation of adhesions. Endometriosis can deposit in many sites including pelvis, bowel, and bladder and as the lesions are oestrogen sensitive, symptoms vary through the menstrual cycle.

History:

The symptoms of endometriosis are varied and can be non-specific. They can range from minimal to debilitating. Endometriosis patients commonly present with severe dysmenorrhea, which can begin prior to menstruation and persist through and beyond. For some, subfertility is the presenting complaint. Endometriosis can also cause chronic pelvic pain and deep dyspareunia, periodic bloating and fatigue. Other symptoms are dependent on location of disease; dyschezia and haematochezia may indicate bowel involvement, and dysuria, haematuria or flank pain can result from urinary system involvement.

A symptom diary may prove useful in identifying symptoms which a patient may not recognise as being related to endometriosis. The impact of endometriosis on the patient's quality of life should be defined to inform any support needed.

Examination:

On examination, the findings in endometriosis are dependent of ectopic tissue and adhesion location. On a pelvic examination, ovarian or ligament endometriosis may be palpable as adnexal masses or nodules. Adhesions may also cause changes of anatomy including fixing the uterus into a retroverted position. On abdominal examination, patients may have masses and generalised tenderness.

Investigations:

In the primary care setting, investigations are not needed to confirm endometriosis and a clinical diagnosis is made before commencing low risk medical treatment.

A transvaginal ultrasound can be used to confirm ovarian endometriomas or deep pelvic involvement and can detect any resulting pelvic immobility. MRI is used to assess the extent of any suspected bladder, bowel, or ureter involvement.

If definitive diagnosis is needed, for example for more invasive management, a diagnostic laparoscopy and biopsy of any 'chocolate cysts', peritoneal deposits or adhesions is indicated.

Management:

Medical management: The first line medical management of endometriosis pain is with hormonal contraceptives and non-steroidal anti-inflammatories. Both combined and progestogen-based contraceptives can be tried and can be used continuously to prolong amenorrhoeic periods.

If hormonal contraceptives and analgesia fail to control pain, GNRH antagonists or agonists can be used to induce a hypo-oestrogenic and therefore temporary menopausal state, reducing endometriosis processes for this time. Use of these drugs is time limited due to menopausal symptoms and osteoporosis risk, and add-on hormones are indicated to reduce these.

Surgical pain management: If medical treatment is insufficient to control pain and fertility is a desired in the future, gynaecologists may offer laparoscopic surgery. Adhesions are divided and visible endometriotic implants can be removed. In deep endometriosis normal anatomy can be restored. However, endometriosis is likely to recur and surgery can contribute to adhesion formation.

If fertility is not desired, a hysterectomy might be considered, with removal of visible peritoneal implants. However, some patients experience symptoms post hysterectomy.

Fertility management: Laparoscopic surgical resection and ablation of endometrial implants can improve fertility as well as pain. Fertility treatments may also be offered earlier to those with a diagnosis of endometriosis than the general population.

Psychological support: Endometriosis can be a life changing chronic condition. It is therefore important to provide psychological support and direct to local support groups and charities.

Patients should be referred to gynaecology service if endometriosis symptoms are severe or persistent despite primary medical treatment or there is suspected involvement of the bladder, bowel, or ureter.

Irregular menstrual bleeding

Vignette

You are a final year medical student working on your GP placement. Karen, a 25-year-old lady, has come in to discuss her irregular periods. Please take a history and offer any examinations you would like to conduct. At 6 minutes, you will receive questions from the examiner.

You have 8 minutes for this station

Patient brief

Presenting complaint:

You are a 28-year-old lady who has been having irregular periods for the past year.

History of presenting complaint:

Your last menstrual period was 3 months ago, and you have only had one other period in the past year. They lasted around 5 days, with no intermenstrual or postcoital bleeding. Your periods are not heavy or painful. You never pass clots, leak, or need to use double protection. Your age of menarche was 13 and your periods used to be on a regular 28-day cycle. You do not have a problem with vaginal dryness or hot flushes and your mother reached menopause aged 55.

You have also noticed that you have gained a bit of weight recently despite unchanged eating or exercise habits, and you do not exercise or diet excessively. You have also been struggling with increased facial hair and mild acne, although this is longstanding. You have not experienced any tremors, hot or cold intolerance or palpitations. You have not experienced any discharge from the nipple. You are otherwise well with no urinary or bowel symptoms, no pain, no fever, no weight loss or night sweats.

Obstetric history:

You have never been pregnant, but you eventually want to start a family with your partner, and are worried that you might be infertile because of your irregular periods.

Gynaecological history:

You are up to date with your cervical smears and they have all been normal.

Sexual history:

You have no dyspareunia, no abnormal vaginal discharge and have never been diagnosed with a sexually transmitted infection. You only use condoms for contraception.

Past medical history:

You have mild asthma, for which you use a salbutamol inhaler as needed. You had a laparoscopic appendicectomy aged 24 and had no issues post operatively.

Past surgical history:

Nil

Drug history:

You are not on any regular medication other than the PRN salbutamol and occasional over-the-counter paracetamol use for headaches. No known drug allergies

Family history:

Your mother had breast cancer aged 62, cured with mastectomy.

Social history:

You are a teacher and live at home with your partner of 3 years. You smoke 10 cigarettes a day and have done for 8 years, and you drink socially on weekends. You are worried that you will not be able to get pregnant and you are also starting to feel self-conscious about the weight gain. You are hoping to get some blood tests to find out why your periods have become irregular.

Examination:

All examination findings are unremarkable.

BMI 25

Questions at 6 minutes:

What are your differential diagnoses?

PCOS, hypothyroidism, pregnancy, stress, excessive exercise, premature ovarian failure, hyperprolactinaemia

What further investigations would you like to conduct?

Pregnancy test, FSH, LH, testosterone, TFTs, serum prolactin

Going with the diagnosis of PCOS, how would you manage this patient?

Lifestyle changes (quitting smoking, weight loss)

Ensure menstrual bleed at least every 3-4 months to reduce the risk of endometrial hyperplasia/cancer (e.g. cyclical COCP, or a course of progesterone every 3-4 months)

Screen for depression

Check BP/lipid profile/HbA1C if indicated

Clomiphene and metformin if trying to get pregnant.

Ovarian drilling as second line it trying to conceive

Mark scheme

Introduces themselves, and confirms patients name and date of birth	/1
Establishes menstrual cycle (how often periods occur, duration, menorrhagia/dysmenorrhoea, age of menarche)	/2
Asks about PCOS symptoms (weight gain, acne, hirsutism, fertility)	/2
Asks about thyroid symptoms (sweating/tremors, hair changes, hot/cold intolerance)	/2
Asks about excessive dieting or exercise	/1
Asks about premature menopause symptoms (hot flushes, night sweats, vaginal dryness)	/1
Asks about symptoms of hyperprolactinaemia (headaches, visual disturbances, nipple discharge)	/1
Screens for systemic symptoms (bowels, bladder, pain, fever) and red flags (weight loss, night sweats)	/2
Asks about obstetric history	/1
Asks about gynaecological history (including cervical smears)	/1
Asks about sexual history, contraception and fertility	/1
Asks about past medical/surgical history	/1
Asks about drug history and allergies	/1
Asks about family history	/1
Asks about social history (occupation, home situation, smoking and drinking)	/1
Explores ideas, concerns and expectations	/1
Offers to examine the patient	/1
Gives sensible differential diagnoses (Polycystic ovarian syndrome, hypothyroid, pregnancy, stress, excessive exercise, premature ovarian failure, hyperprolactinaemia)	/2
Offers sensible investigations (Pregnancy test, FSH, LH, testosterone, TFTs, serum prolactin, pelvic ultrasound)	/2
Establishes a structured management plan:	/3

-Lifestyle changes: quitting smoking, weight loss -Screen for depression -Can consider screening BP/lipid profile/HbA1C -Ensure menstrual bleed at least every 3-4 months: COCP, cyclical progesterone, POP, Mirena, Depo-Provera -Clomiphene or Metformin if trying to get pregnant -Surgical management: Ovarian drilling	
Shows empathy and good patient manner in consultation	/2

Additional information

Polycystic ovarian syndrome (PCOS) is an heterogenous endocrine disorder that is thought to be a combination of genetic and environmental factors. It is usually diagnosed by using the Rotterdam Criteria; this is the presence of two of the three criteria: hyperandrogenism, irregular/absent ovulation and polycystic ovaries on ultrasound (>12 follicles of 2-9mm in diameter).

Whilst the exact aetiology is unknown, the ovaries and adrenals are stimulated to produce excessive amounts of androgenic hormones, likely due to excess LH release from the anterior pituitary and/or hyperinsulinemia. This that causes the development of multiple follicles that do not fully mature for ovulation. This excess testosterone also causes the other symptoms such as acne and hirsutism.

Patients with PCOS have an increased risk of cardiovascular disease and diabetes, and can often have a high BMI, and as such should be monitored for these. Furthermore, high levels of oestrogen in the condition can cause endometrial hyperplasia and increased risk of endometrial cancer.

PCOS can also increase risk for subfertility.

These symptoms can lead to low mood or depression, so screening for depression is also vital for management.

Examination

General examination can be useful to pick up features such as acne, hirsutism and acanthosis nigricans, alongside considering other differential diagnoses (particularly symptoms of thyroid disease). Abdominal examination may be normal; pelvic examination could demonstrate enlarged ovaries.

Investigations

- Pregnancy test – very important to rule out with oligo/amenorrhoea
- FSH/LH levels – if persistently elevated, could indicate premature ovarian failure. In PCOS, LH is usually raised more than FSH.
- Testosterone – levels raised in PCOS
- Thyroid function tests – to rule out thyroid disease
- Serum prolactin – to rule out hyperprolactinaemia
- Pelvis ultrasound – usually show a 'string of pearls' appearance

Management

Conservative:

Offer advice on lifestyle changes including losing weight, exercising, stopping smoking and reducing alcohol intake.

Medical

It is vital to ensure that women with PCOS have menstrual bleeds every 3-4 months to reduce the risk of endometrial hyperplasia and cancer. This can be achieved using hormonal contraception (cyclical COCP, POP, Depo-Provera, Implant, Mirena coil) or with cyclical progesterone therapy. In particular, the COCP can bring down levels of androgens, thus improving the symptoms of PCOS (acne, hirsutism).

As PCOS patients have a higher risk of metabolic syndrome, it is important to screen for BP/lipid profile/HbA1C.

Clomiphene and metformin can be used if the patient is trying to get pregnant, however there is a risk of ovarian hyperstimulation from fertility medications.

Surgical:

Ovarian drilling – this is a surgical technique of puncturing membranes of the ovary with a laser or needle and can be done laparoscopically. It is thought to reduce the level of androgens produced by the ovaries and can be especially useful in improving fertility.

Menorrhagia

Vignette

You are a final year medical student working on your GP placement. Please take a history from this 32-year-old lady with heavy menstrual bleeds.

Patient brief

HPC: You are Angela Jones, a 32-year-old librarian who has been suffering with heavy periods over the last 2 years. You have regular cycles occurring every 28 days and lasting 6 days with no intermenstrual or postcoital bleeding. The bleeding is heavier on the first two days of the cycle where you soak 10-15 pads per day with clots and require double protection. Your periods are not too painful. You find it difficult to go to work on the first two days of your period as the bleeding is too heavy. You have no deep dyspareunia and have never had a sexually transmitted infection. You have no symptoms of hypothyroidism.

You have a regular sexual partner and use condoms for contraception. You last had a sexual health check two years ago which was normal. You have regular smear tests, which have all been normal. You have previously had one medical termination of pregnancy 5 years ago. No other pregnancies. You have no abnormal discharge.

Past medical History: Nil

Drug History: Nil. NKDA

Family History: Nil

Social History: Non-smoker. Occasional alcohol.

Examiner to ask student:

1) Potential causes of menorrhagia
2) Investigations in this case
3) First line management options

Mark Scheme

Item	Mark
Introduces themselves	/1
Confirms name, age, occupation	/2
History of presenting complaint, including: • Assessment of severity of symptoms • Effect on quality of life	/5
Previous gynaecological history, including: • Menstrual – LMP, regularity of cycles, dyspareunia, IMB/PCB • Smears – last smear and results • Sexual history – including contraception and previous STIs	/4
Symptoms of hypothyroid as potential cause	/2
Previous obstetric history	/1
Medical history	/1
Drug history (including contraception)	/1
Family history	/1
Social history	/1
Possible causes for menorrhagia • Uterine fibroids • Endometrial polyp • Dysfunctional uterine bleeding	/2
Investigations • FBC • Thyroid function tests if signs or symptoms • Ultrasound if suggestion of structural/histological abnormality	/2
First line management options • First line: Mirena coil if >12 months use is anticipated • Second line: Tranexamic acid/COCP/NSAIDs	/2
Examiners and patients score	/5
Overall	/30

Additional information

Menorrhagia is classically defined as menstruation which is greater than 80 ml per cycle. However menstrual blood volume is impractical to measure, therefore clinically menorrhagia is a subjectively excessive volume or length of menstrual bleeding, affecting the patient's quality of life. Menorrhagia is very common, with prevalence increasing with age.

Menorrhagia can cause anaemia and symptoms can include fatigue and dizziness. Menorrhagia often negatively affects the quality of many aspects of a woman's life. A thorough history and examination should be taken to screen for the characteristics and signs of common causes of menorrhagia.

Aetiology:

The International Federation of Gynaecology and Obstetrics (FIGO) describes the PALM-COEIN system to categorise causes of abnormal intrauterine bleeding:

Endometrial structural causes: Polyps, adenomyosis, (submucosal) leiomyomas, malignancy/hyperplasia (PALM)

Non-structural causes: coagulopathy, ovulatory dysfunction, endometrial, iatrogenic, not yet classified (COEIN)

Coagulopathy can cause menorrhagia and patients may also present with easy bruising, prolonged mucosal bleeding and have often had menorrhagia since the onset of menstruation.

Ovulatory dysfunction can cause menorrhagia, and is often associated with irregular cycle length. A lack of ovulation results in no luteinising hormone surge or progesterone production, leading to unopposed oestrogen stimulation of the endometrium, and excessive endometrial growth and bleeding. Anovulation causes include polycystic ovarian syndrome and hypothyroidism.

Iatrogenic causes of menorrhagia include copper intrauterine devices, anticoagulation and systemic corticosteroid therapy.

In the majority of cases, menorrhagia is idiopathic, termed **dysfunctional uterine bleeding.**

Investigations:

All women of reproductive age should have a pregnancy urine test to ensure there is no pregnancy involved.

Full blood count is necessary for diagnosis of anaemia caused by the menorrhagia. The remaining investigations are dependent on history and examination to diagnose causative disorders, for example thyroid function tests and coagulation screen. Women who have a history or examination suggestive of structural abnormalities should receive ultrasound or hysteroscopic imaging.

Management:

The choice of management is based on severity of symptoms and desire for fertility. In addition, if there is a known cause for menorrhagia, this can be directly treated.

Medical Management:

The levonorgestrel intrauterine contraceptive system (Mirena coil) is offered first line for menorrhagia and suppresses endometrial proliferation. Alternatively, combined oral contraceptive or cyclical oral progestogens can be trialled.

Tranexamic acid and non-steroidal anti-inflammatory drugs (mefenamic acid, naproxen and ibuprofen) can be offered as an adjunct or alternative if fertility is desired and should be taken during menstrual bleeds only.

Surgical Management:

Surgical management options include hysteroscopic resection of submucosal fibroids, abdominal myomectomy, uterine artery embolization, endometrial ablation, and hysterectomy. Hysterectomy is the only option to definitively manage menorrhagia, however, use in menorrhagia management has greatly decreased since the introduction of less invasive options.

Ovarian Torsion

Vignette

You are the gynaecology Foundation year 2 doctor and have been asked to see 25-year-old Cathy, who has presented with severe pelvic pain. Please take a short history and describe the examinations you would like to do. You will then be asked questions about the case.

Patient Brief

Presenting Complaint:

You are experiencing severe and constant right sided iliac fossa pain, which started suddenly 1 hour ago whilst you were at work. You have vomited three times since then and feel very nauseous and lightheaded 'due to the pain'. You have had no vaginal bleeding or change in discharge. You have had no recent change of bowel habit, bladder and no previous similar episodes.

Gynaecological history:

You have had no previous pregnancies. Your periods are normally every 30 days and you bleed 'fairly heavily' for five days. Your last menstrual period started 16 days ago. You have used the combined oral contraceptive pill since you were 17 years old. You last had STI screening last year which was negative and have had several sexual partners since then, although always used condoms. You have yet to have your first smear test.

Past medical and surgical history:

You have no medical problems and have had a previous appendicectomy.

Social history: You smoke occasionally and drink around 1.5 bottles of wine a week. You work in marketing.

Family history: Nil

On examination:

Observations:

Heart rate: 105 beats per minute Blood pressure: 85/60mm/hg

Respiratory rate: 16 breaths per minute Oxygen saturation: 99% on room air

Temperature: 37.2°c

Abdominal examination: Generalised abdominal tenderness, which is severe in right iliac fossa with moderate guarding, there are no palpable masses or scars.

Pelvic examination: Normal external genitalia. Normal sized anteverted uterus. Right adnexal tenderness with no cervical excitation. No bleeding or discharge visible on speculum examination.

Questions

1. **List your differentials for this case**
2. **Describe examinations you would like to carry out**

Urine dip pregnancy test: negative

Urine dip: negative for all

Pelvic ultrasound: enlarged right ovary with reduced vascularity on doppler.

Point of care haemoglobin test: 120mg/

Blood tests: Results pending

High vaginal swab: Results pending

3. **What is your primary diagnosis?**
4. **How would you manage ovarian torsion?**
5. **Who is at risk of ovarian torsion?**

Mark scheme

Introduces self and confirms patient identity	/1
Defines presenting complaint including: • Associated urinary or bowel symptoms	/4
Gynaecological and obstetric history including: • Menstrual history • Sexual health history	/2 /1 /1
Family history	/1
Social history	/1
Focused and concise history	/1
Examination • Observations • Abdominal examination • Pelvic examination	/3
Differential diagnoses, at least four of: • Ovarian torsion, ovarian cyst rupture, ovulation pain, pyelonephritis, renal colic, mesenteric adenitis, pelvic inflammatory disease	/4
Investigations, at least three of: • Urine β-hcg, urine dipstick, group & save, full blood count, CRP, vaginal swabs, pelvic ultrasound	/3
Management • Analgesia and stabilisation if required • Surgical management including detorsion or ovarian cystectomy	/4

Risk factors • ovarian masses, pregnancy, previous tubal ligation, ovulation induction	/2
Answers questions with clear structure and classification	/2
Total	/30

Additional information

A focused history, physical examination and observations are needed to quickly assess a presentation of acute pelvic pain to identify the need for urgent stabilisation or management. There is a wide range of causes for acute pelvic pain; differential diagnosis should consider the following:

Urinary system: Urinary Tract Infection, ureteric colic

Colorectal system: Appendicitis, bowel obstruction, diverticulitis, bowl perforation.

Gynaecological system: Ovarian cyst rupture or haemorrhage, ovarian torsion, ovulation pain, ectopic pregnancy, pelvic inflammatory disease, uterine fibroid degeneration.

Ovarian torsion:

Ovarian torsion is the rotation of an ovary and fallopian tubes on their ligamentous support, compromising venous and lymphatic outflow, and causing ovarian oedema and vascular compression. Early diagnosis and management are crucial to preserve ovarian function, as complete torsion quickly leads to ischaemia and infarction. Torsion may become complicated with peritonitis and induce pelvic adhesions. Chronic adnexal torsion can result in hydrosalpinx.

Ovarian torsion presents as acute severe pelvic pain, which is often unilateral, and commonly with nausea and vomiting. On abdominal examination, patients can have generalised tenderness, localised guarding and rebound tenderness. On vaginal examination, there may be a palpable adnexal mass, adnexal tenderness or cervical excitation. Patients may also have low grade pyrexia and become systemically unwell, with metabolic acidosis.

Enlarged ovaries are at increased risk of torsion, including due to functional, dermoid and paraovarian cysts, ovarian malignancy and in patients undergoing ovulation induction for fertility treatment. Additionally, a history of tubal sterilisation and current pregnancy both increase the risk of torsion.

Investigations:

Urine pregnancy testing should be carried out on all women of reproductive age presenting with abdominal pain to exclude ectopic pregnancy. Urine dipstick testing would detect no abnormalities in ovarian torsion unless there is coexisting urinary tract infection or calculi. Ovarian torsion can cause leucocytosis and elevated C-reactive protein, however if severe anaemia is present an alternate diagnosis causing haemorrhage should be considered. If the patient is postmenopausal, serum Ca-125 levels should be taken because ovarian malignancy increases risk of torsion. Vaginal swabs should be taken to rule out coexisting or alternate diagnosis of pelvic inflammatory disease.

Pelvic ultrasound is used for fast and detailed visualisation of ovaries, which may appear enlarged, greater than 4cm, due to oedema and haemorrhage. Free pelvic fluid, a 'whirlpool' twisted pedicle and underlying ovarian lesion may also be visible. If available, Doppler studies can show reduced or absent vascularity. Ultrasound findings in torsion are highly dynamic, advanced torsion may appear as a solid mass with areas of haemorrhage and necrosis. Normal ultrasound does not rule out torsion.

Although investigations strengthen suspicion, decision for management should be clinical. Torsion can only be confirmed with direct visualisation at surgery for definitive diagnosis.

<u>Management:</u>

After the patient is stabilised and analgesia is started, urgent surgery should be organised to prevent irreversible ovarian necrosis and further complications. The surgical management of ovarian torsion is guided by the patient's menopausal status, background of ovarian pathology and fertility desires. Younger women and those who have not completed their family should be offered detorsion, to aim to preserve ovarian function and fertility. Additionally, if there is 'non-functional' ovarian cyst visible, cystectomy should be carried out. For postmenopausal women, those who do not desire fertility, and if there is suspected malignancy, salpingo-oophorectomy may be organised.

Overactive Bladder Syndrome

Vignette

You are a Foundation year 2 Doctor in a GP surgery. 60-year-old Nancy has come in to discuss the recent changes in her urinary habit. Please take a history and explain suitable investigations and treatment options.

Patient brief

Presenting complaint- You have been experiencing uncontrollable urges to urinate for the past year, which cause you to run to the toilet. In the past 3 months you have had many episodes where you have not been able to get to the toilet in time and have leaked, last week three times.

History of presenting complaint- There is no predictability to the urges, and they are not associated with exertion, coughing or sneezing. It significantly disrupts your activities as you are anxious to make sure you are always near a toilet. The urge to urinate happens around 12 times a day and you wake about twice on average per night to urinate. You wear incontinence pads when you go for a long day out. Your urine is normal in appearance and smell and you do not experience burning on passing urine.

Obstetric history- You have had 3 children born by vaginal delivery; you had an episiotomy which healed well during your first labour. You had one miscarriage at 11 weeks and have had no termination of pregnancies.

Gynaecological history- You had your last menstrual period 8 years ago and have not needed hormone replacement therapy. All your smears have been normal. Your menstrual periods lasted 27 days on average and you bled for 5 days, with no menorrhagia or dysmenorrhea.

Past medical history- You have hypertension which is well treated and seasonal Hay fever. You have had no previous surgery or any neurological disease.

Sexual history- Sex has become increasingly more painful in last 5 years and you sometimes get postcoital bleeding. You are married, with no other current sexual partners apart from your husband.

Family history- No relevant family history

Drug history- Ramipril for hypertension. You sometimes take cetirizine, an antihistamine for allergies.

Allergies- No drug allergies

Social history- You are a retired nurse and live at home with your husband. You drink lots of water and coffee, and alcohol 'on weekends' only. You are a non-smoker. You used to enjoy regular exercise classes but have not been in last 2 months as are afraid of not being able to get to the toilet in time, you have put on 5kg in this time period which you are very upset about. You have also become quite low recently as have been staying at home and avoiding social events.

Mark scheme

Introduces themselves and confirms patient identity	/1
Defines presenting complaint • Screens for stress incontinence, including worsening with sneezing, laughing and coughing • Screens for urge incontinence, including frequency, nocturia and urgency • Screens for outflow obstruction, including hesitancy, poor stream, terminal dribbling • Screens for urinary tract infection, including frothy, foul smelling urine, dysuria and fevers • Systems review- for malignancy symptoms including weight loss and hematuria	/1 /2 /2 /1 /1 /1
Asks about obstetric and gynaecological history • Including menopause and hormone replacement therapy	/3 /1
Past medical and surgical history Family history Drug history	/2 /1 /1
Fluid intake history, including volume of fluid intake, caffeinated drinks	/2
Asks questions to quantify effect on quality of life, at least 2 of • Sleep, Sexual function, Independence, Mood	/2
• Offers appropriate examination and investigations, including abdominal and pelvic examination, urine dip and bladder diary	/2
Gives sensible differentials. Offers sensible management plan, starting with conservative options • Lifestyle changes- caffeine or fluid reduction, weight loss • Therapies- bladder retraining program • Medical management- muscarinic anticholinergic, intravaginal oestrogens	/2 /3

• Invasive- Botox A injection if detrusor overactivity, nerve stimulation	
Shows empathy and good patient manner in consultation	/2
Total	/30

Additional information

Overactive bladder syndrome is characterised by increased urgency, frequency and nocturia which may or may not result in incontinence. In most this is because of detrusor muscle overactivity. It is more common in older women with prolapse and who have had pelvic surgery. Neurological conditions can contribute to bladder overactivity, including multiple sclerosis, spinal cord injury and Parkinson's disease. Multiple comorbidities can worsen the burden for example heart failure, type 2 diabetes, and urinary tract infections.

Stress incontinence:

In stress incontinence, leaks occur after increases in intra-abdominal pressure, such as exertion, sneezing and coughing. It is caused by poor support of bladder and urethra by pelvic floor musculature. Risk factors include high parity, vaginal deliveries and episiotomies as well as obesity.

Stress and urgency incontinence can coexist- termed 'mixed incontinence'

Overflow incontinence:

Overflow incontinence is urinary leakage from an overdistended bladder in chronic urinary retention.

Triggers and effect on life:

- Medications can also cause or exacerbate incontinence. Urinary retention and thereby overflow incontinence can be worsened by drugs such as anticholinergics, antidepressants, antihistamines, benzodiazepines, antipsychotics and calcium channel blockers. By contrast, parasympathomimetic can worsen detrusor overactivity and urge incontinence. Diuretics greatly increase urine output.

- History of fluid intake is important as caffeinated, acidic and alcoholic drinks can exacerbate urge incontinence. Increased fluid intake can increase the burden of the condition.
- Urinary incontinence and overactive bladder syndrome can have a major impact on quality of life; it is very important to assess the psychosocial impact it may be having; particularly for sexual, sleep, financial or mobility problems.

Examination:

General examination is indicated, for detection of relevant comorbidities including neurological disorders. Assess for any abdominal mass including faecal loading as this can increase intraabdominal pressure and distort normal micturition. Pelvic examination for evidence of any prolapse, masses, or vaginal atrophy and to assess pelvic floor muscle strength digitally.

Investigations:

- Urine dipstick to test for concurrent urinary tract infection and microscopic haematuria.
- Post void residual bladder scan if overflow incontinence suspected.
- Urea and electrolytes in overflow incontinence to quantify renal damage.
- A bladder diary detailing fluid intake, episodes of urgency and incontinence, including triggers and use of pads
- Urodynamic testing in resistant cases of incontinence before consideration of invasive therapy.

Treatment for overactive bladder and urge incontinence:

- Conservative: Recommend weight loss for those with a BMI over 30 and to reduce excessive fluid and caffeine intake.
- Therapies: Bladder retraining, gradually increasing periods between urination can ease bladder overactivity
- Medical: Antimuscarinic drugs inhibit bladder contractions, however may have adverse effects in those with cognitive impairment. Vaginal oestrogen may also be useful.

- Invasive: Botulinum toxin type A injection into bladder wall can inhibit detrusor overactivity. Neuromodulation via courses of Posterial Tibial or Sacral Nerve Stimulation can also be considered.

Treatment for stress incontinence

- Conservative: Recommend weight loss for those with a BMI over 30. Treat chronic constipation and cough as these may be aggravating factors.
- Therapies: Pelvic floor exercises can help strengthen the pelvic floor and reduce symptoms of stress incontinence.
- Invasive: Tension Free Vaginal Tape (TVT), although this is used less frequently now as it involves use of mesh. Colposuspension can be used to support the urethra (laparoscopically or open). Bulking agents can also be injected around the bladder entrance to keep it closed.

Postmenopausal Bleeding

Vignette

You are a medical student on your GP placement. You have been asked to see Pamela Gordon, a 55-year-old woman who has noticed new vaginal bleeding. Explain to the woman what the potential differential diagnoses are and what further investigations and management you will perform.

Patient Brief

Presenting Complaint:
You introduce yourself (Pamela Gordon, 25/7/65) and explain that your period has returned despite thinking you had already gone through menopause.

History of Presenting Complaint:
The bleeding started 4 days ago with spotting but for the past 2 days, it has been heavier like a period. You are having to use sanitary towels and you have had to change your pad twice today and yesterday. There are no clots and you have not had any flooding. This is your first episode of this type of bleeding.

You have never had any abnormal vaginal bleeding and you do not have any abnormal vaginal discharge. You have noticed your vagina has actually become quite dry and sore for the past year which makes sometimes makes sex painful. You do not have any abdominal or pelvic pain, or distension. You have had ongoing "leaking" since giving birth, but you have no other urinary symptoms. You have IBS so often have irregular bowel habits and bloating. You have been getting more tired recently, but you suspect this is due to getting older. You have no night sweats, fevers or loss of appetite. In fact, you have probably gained more weight since retiring.

The bleeding has not had a significant impact on your life, but it is an inconvenience as you thought you did not have to have periods anymore!

Obstetric and Gynaecological History:
You cannot remember the exact date of your last menstrual period, but they stopped two years ago, which is when you thought you went through the menopause. Prior to this, they had become more and more infrequent. You do not have any hot flushes, but you have vaginal dryness. Your cervical smears are normal and up to date, and you have never been checked for STIs.

You have been pregnant once and gave birth by normal vaginal delivery in 1999. You have never had any miscarriages or terminations. You are sexually active with your husband of 36 years and you are not using any contraception. He has never been checked for STIs either.

Past Medical and Surgical History:
You have no past medical or surgical history.

Drug History and Allergies:

You do not take any medication and you have no known drug allergies.

Family History:
Your sister and aunt had breast cancer, and your grandfather died of colorectal cancer.

Social History:
You are a retired teacher and you live in a house with your husband. You manage well independently, and your son and his family regularly visit. You have never smoked, occasionally drink on special occasions and have never taken recreational drugs.

Ideas, Concerns and Expectations:
You are not particularly concerned about this bleeding, but you thought you should get it checked out as it is unusual.

The examiner will now ask the candidate some questions.

1) What examinations and investigations should be undertaken?
2) What is the most important differential diagnoses and its subsequent management?

Mark Scheme

Item	Mark
Introduces self with full name and role	/1
Confirms patient's identity	/1
Asks an open question to begin the consultation	/1
Enquires about the characteristics of the bleeding • Onset and duration • Progression • Intermittent or continuous • Amount of blood loss: number of sanitary towels/tampons, clots, flooding • Exacerbating and relieving factors • Previous episodes • Relation to menstrual cycle	/2
Enquires about associated symptoms such as: • Abnormal vaginal bleeding: post-coital, intermenstrual, menorrhagia, dysmenorrhoea • Abnormal vaginal discharge • Abdominal or pelvic pain • Abdominal distension • Genital skin changes, itching or soreness • Dyspareunia • Change in urinary symptoms: frequency, urgency and dysuria • Change in bowel habits • General malaise, night sweats, fever, loss of appetite or unintentional weight loss • Symptoms of anaemia: dizziness, fatigue, breathlessness, chest pain, palpitations	/2
Enquires about effect on life	/2
Takes a gynaecological history:	/2

• Date of last menstrual period • Duration and frequency of periods • Abnormal vaginal bleeding • Age at menarche • Age at menopause • Menopausal symptoms: hot flushes, vaginal dryness • Cervical screening history: last checked, results, any treatment required • STI history: last checked, results, any treatment required	
Takes an obstetric history: • Any previous or current pregnancies • Any miscarriages or terminations	/1
Takes a sexual history: • Enquires if sexually active and with whom • Sensitively enquires about consent • Establishes whether regular or casual partner • Use of contraception • Enquires about partner's STI history	/1
Enquires about past medical and surgical history: • Migraine with aura, venous thromboembolism, breast cancer or bleeding disorders	/1
Enquires about drug history and allergies: • HRT, tamoxifen, anticoagulants	/1
Enquires about family history: • Ovarian, endometrial or breast cancer • Bleeding disorders • Venous thromboembolism	/1
Enquires about social history • Student or employment status	/1

• Living arrangements • Smoking, alcohol and use of recreational drugs	
Gains patient's ideas, concerns, and expectations	/2
Explains to the patient that there are a number of differential diagnoses, and these include endometrial cancer and vagina atrophy. 10% of women with postmenopausal bleeding will have endometrial cancer.	/2
Further investigations aim to identify those women with potential pre-cancer or cancer of the endometrium, so that if found, treatment can be initiated in the early stages. Investigations include FBC and transvaginal and abdominal ultrasound. If the ultrasound shows raised endometrial thickness, then the patient will need a hysteroscopy and biopsy (camera test to look at the lining of the womb and take a sample for diagnosis)	/3
Explains that a 2 week wait referral will be made to gynaecology. Reassures patient that this does not mean she has cancer but is a way of expediting investigations so that cases of cancer can be picked up early where they are more amenable to treatment.	/2
Chunks and checks	/1
Provides a leaflet	/1
Appropriately closes the consultation and thanks the patient	/1
Behaves in a professional manner	/1
Total	/30

Additional Information

Menopause is typically defined as when a woman has not had a period for more than 12 months. This usually happens in a woman's late 40s or early 50s, although this can happen earlier or later in life. Any bleeding following this is defined as postmenopausal bleeding and must be investigated.

Differential Diagnosis

- Atrophic vaginitis
  - due to reduced oestrogen levels
  - thin friable vaginal wall with contact bleeding on speculum examination
  - can be managed with topical or systemic oestrogens
- Endometrial atrophy
  - due to reduced oestrogen levels
  - can be managed conservatively, or with oestrogen cream or pessaries
- Cervical or endometrial polyps
  - can be removed during hysteroscopy
- Endometrial hyperplasia
  - can be managed conservatively, with progestogens or surgery
- HRT
  - can change or stop treatment
- Cervical cancer
- Endometrial cancer
- Vaginal cancer
- Uterine cancer

Risk Factors for Endometrial Cancer

- Nulliparity
- Early menarche
- Late menopause
- Unopposed oestrogen therapy
- Obesity
- Diabetes mellitus
- Tamoxifen
- Atypical endometrial hyperplasia

Referral Pathway for Endometrial Cancer

Urgent 2 week wait referral if more than 55 years old with postmenopausal bleeding.

Consider an urgent 2 week wait referral if less than 55 years old with postmenopausal bleeding.

In these patients, transvaginal ultrasound is the appropriate first-line procedure to identify which women with postmenopausal bleeding are at higher risk of endometrial cancer. The mean endometrial thickness in postmenopausal women is much thinner than in pre-menopausal women. Thickening of the endometrium may indicate the presence of pathology. In general, the thicker the endometrium, the higher the likelihood of endometrial cancer being present. Most hospitals use a cut-off of 4-5mm, with thickening above this warranting a hysteroscopy and biopsy. If the endometrial thickness is less than 4-5mm, and the bleeding was one-off, a woman can be reassured that likelihood of endometrial cancer is low. If the endometrial thickness is less than 4-5mm, but bleeding is recurrent, a hysteroscopy and biopsy will usually be recommended.

Termination of pregnancy

Vignette

You are a junior doctor working in a termination of pregnancy clinic. Tonia Steel, an 18-year-old girl, has come in to discuss termination of pregnancy. Please take a short history and counsel her on her options, answering any questions she may have.

You have 8 minutes for this station.

Patient brief

Presenting complaint:

You are Tonia Steel, an 18-year-old girl who has presented to her local termination of pregnancy clinic to discuss abortion.

History of presenting complaint:

You have been with your current partner for a year. He is in your year at school and all sexual activity has been consensual. You have been using 'pulling out' as your form of contraception, but you have been meaning to use proper contraception. You realised you missed your last period, and decided to take a pregnancy test, which was positive.

You have discussed the pregnancy with your partner. As you will both be starting university next month, you agree that you are not ready to be parents. You have also told your sister, who has been very supportive, but strongly do not want your parents to know about this.

You have read a bit about termination of pregnancy and are worried about the pain it may cause. You are otherwise well and asymptomatic.

Obstetric history:

You had never been pregnant before.

Gynaecological history:

You have regular periods on a 30-day cycle, which last 7 days and are not heavy or painful. Your last menstrual period started 8 weeks ago. You never leak, pass clots, or have to use double protection. You do not get postcoital bleeding or intermenstrual bleeding. You have not started having cervical smears yet. Your age of menarche was 16.

Sexual history:

You only have sex with men and have only ever been with your current partner, who is from the UK. You have never been diagnosed with a sexually transmitted infection, and your last sexual health screen was 1 year ago, which was negative. You do not use any regular form of contraception.

Past medical history:

No other medical conditions.

Past surgical history:

No previous surgery.

Drug history:

You do not take any regular medications.

Family history:

Your mother had breast cancer aged 50 – she had a mastectomy and is now in remission.

Social history:

You have just finished school and are about to start university. You are happy in your relationship but worried about the stress of starting university and know you could not cope with having a baby. You have been accompanied by your partner, who is very supportive of your decision, but have not told your parents.

You do not smoke and drink a few drinks on nights out on the weekends. You occasionally smoke cannabis.

Questions to ask:

What are my options at this stage (8 weeks)?

At this stage, express that you would like to try a medical termination

What will I experience with a medical termination?

What are the risks of a medical termination?

What is the latest stage in pregnancy that I can have a termination?

Can doctors refuse to perform terminations?

Mark scheme

Introduces themselves, and confirms patients name and date of birth	/1
Discusses doctor-patient confidentiality	/1
Asks when the patient started their last menstrual period, to ascertain how many weeks pregnant she is	/1
Offers a pregnancy test in the clinic to confirm pregnancy	/1
Explores the reasons behind wanting a termination of pregnancy	/1
Establishes what support the patient has, and who she has discussed this decision with	/1
Performs a risk assessment to rule out partner violence or reproductive coercion	/1
Discusses the use of contraception	/1
Takes a obstetric history	/1
Takes a gynaecological history	/1
Takes a sexual history	/1
Takes a past medical and surgical history	/1
Takes a drug history, including allergies	/1
Asks about family history	/1
Asks about social history (occupation, home situation, smoking and drinking)	/1
Ideas, concerns and expectations	/1
Discusses options of not terminating the pregnancy (e.g. adoption, receiving additional help etc)	/1
Discusses medical termination (mifepristone tablet followed by misoprostol a few days later)	/1
Discusses surgical termination (an operation requiring either local or general anaesthetic, and using instruments to manually remove the pregnancy from the womb)	/1
Advises that after a medical termination, the patient may experience pain and bleeding, and advises regular analgesia and wearing sanitary towels, rather than tampons.	/1

Also advises on red flag symptoms (fever, abnormal discharge, ongoing pain or uncontrolled bleeding)	/1
Advises on the risks of a medical termination (incomplete abortion that may then need surgery, prolonged heavy bleeding, uterine perforation, and infection)	/1
Advises that terminations are usually only carried out until 24 weeks, unless there is a risk to life, when it may be carried out later	/1
Advises that while a doctor may decline performing a termination due to personal beliefs, he/she would have an obligation to refer to another clinician who would help	/1
Asks if the patient understands the information given to her, and offers an opportunity to ask any further questions	/1
Offers written information to the patient	/1
Books the patient in for an appointment to perform the procedure, and advises her to bring a friend or family member with her	/1
Books the patient in for an appointment to discuss contraception	/1
Shows empathy and good patient manner in consultation	/2
Total	/30

Additional information

Termination of pregnancy can be a controversial subject. As a doctor, you have the right to refuse to take part in a termination if you conscientiously object. However, your views must never prejudice care, and as such, you must then refer to another practitioner who can help without delay.

Indications

There are several indications for termination of pregnancy, as laid out in the 1967 Abortion Act:

- Continuing the pregnancy would involve a serious risk to maternal life, greater than inf the pregnancy was terminated
- Terminating the pregnancy would be necessary to prevent serious physical or mental health condition to the pregnant woman, or any existing children
- The pregnancy has not exceeded 24 weeks
- The child would be at serious risk of mental or physical handicap if born

Note that **two** registered medical practitioners must be involved in the decision process to ensure the legal grounds are met.

Before a termination

It is always important to perform a pregnancy test +/- a dating ultrasound scan prior to performing a termination.

As detailed in the scenario, it is also important to counsel the patient well. Ask about her thoughts, who she has discussed it with, counsel her on her options and give her time to make a decision.

When she has decided, yourself and another registered practitioner must sign an HS1 form and arrange the termination.

It is also important to discuss contraception early on, and after the procedure, to avoid a further unplanned pregnancy. Long-acting reversible contraception such as the Copper or Mirena coil, Implant may be inserted at the time of the termination of pregnancy.

Medical termination

Medical terminations are usually used up to 10 weeks. Initially an oral dose of mifepristone is given, this is an antiprogesterone that prevents the pregnancy progressing. In the following days, this would be followed by a single dose of misoprostol (either oral or vaginal) – this is a prostaglandin that softens and dilates the cervix and causes uterine contraction, pushing any pregnancy tissue out. Up until 24 weeks, medical terminations may still be used, but would likely need multiple doses of the prostaglandin.

There are also several contraindications to medical termination, including a confirmed or suspected ectopic pregnancy, an IUD (intrauterine device) in situ, long term steroid therapy, chronic adrenal failure, anticoagulant therapy, and a known allergy to any of the agents used.

Whilst medical termination is a relatively safe procedure, it is important to discuss the risks – primary that of an incomplete abortion (that may then need surgery), prolonged bleeding, uterine perforation (particularly later in pregnancy), and infection.

Surgical termination

There are two main methods of surgical termination:

Vacuum or suction aspiration: this can be used up to 14 weeks of pregnancy, and involves a suction tube being inserted into the uterus to gently remove the pregnancy. Misoprostol may be given prior to the procedure to soften the cervix, and the procedure can be done under local or general anaesthetic. It is a quick, day case procedure, lasting 5-10 minutes.

Dilatation and evacuation: this is used later in pregnancy, from 14-24 weeks. A speculum is inserted into the vagina, and dilators may be applied to open the cervix. Small forceps are then inserted into the uterus to remove the pregnancy. The procedure is again short, lasting 10-20 minutes, but has a higher rate of using general anaesthetic.

The risks of surgical terminations are similar, including bleeding, infection, uterine perforation, and damage to the external cervical os.

Care after termination

As well as bleeding and pain, is important to advise patients that after termination (particularly medical terminations) that they may continue to experience nausea, vomiting, dizziness and diarrhoea, although these symptoms should be short lived. With surgical terminations, it is important to discuss the effects of anaesthesia and advise patients not to drive after a procedure. Red flag symptoms must also be highlighted, including fever, abnormal discharge, ongoing pain, or uncontrolled bleeding.

Over the counter painkillers, including paracetamol and ibuprofen are often recommended. Women should also use sanitary pads for any post-procedure bleeding as opposed to tampons. Women can start having sex as soon as they feel comfortable, although if they do not want to get pregnant again then it is important to discuss contraception.

Uterine Prolapse

Vignette

You are an FY2 working at a GP practice. You have been asked to see Ameena Khan, a 57-year-old lady, who has been complaining of lower abdominal discomfort. Please take a history.

You have 7 minutes then the examiner will ask you some questions.

Patient Brief

Presenting Complaint:
You introduce yourself (Ameena Khan, 10/12/63) and explain that you have had some lower abdominal discomfort for the past few months.

History of Presenting Complaint:
You first noticed this discomfort 3 months ago, but It has gotten worse in the past month. It is a constant dragging sensation and it sometimes feels like you are sitting on a ball. You have started having back pain too. You have never had these symptoms before, and they are constant. You are starting to feel low as the heaviness is stopping you from doing things.

You have always leaked urine since giving birth, but you do not have any bowel symptoms. You have recently had some discomfort during sexual intercourse, but this may be due to vaginal dryness since going through menopause. You have never had any abnormal vaginal bleeding and you have not noticed your tummy getting bigger. You feel tired because of this discomfort and pain but you otherwise feel well.

Obstetric and Gynaecological History:
You have 4 children who were all delivered normally. These were in 1983, 1985, 1990 and 1992. You had a miscarriage in 1989. You cannot recall the date of your last menstrual period, but you went through menopause 5 years ago. You have not had any abnormal vaginal bleeding and you first started having periods at 13 years old. You occasionally have hot flushes and you have vaginal dryness. Your cervical smears are up to date and have always been normal.

Sexual History:
You are sexually active with your husband and you do not use contraception anymore. You and your partner have never been checked for STIs.

Past Medical and Surgical History:
You have diabetes and high blood pressure.

Drug History and Allergies:
You take metformin and ramipril, and you have no known drug allergies.

Family History:
Many of your family members have diabetes and high blood pressure.

Social History:
You are a housewife, and you live with your husband and your youngest son. You have never smoked, drunk alcohol or taken any recreational drugs.

Ideas, Concerns and Expectations:
You do not know what is causing these symptoms, but you want to fix this issue as you are usually very independent.

The examiner will now ask the candidate some questions.

1) What is the most likely diagnoses?
2) What are the next steps?

Mark Scheme

Introduces self with full name and role	/1
Confirms patient's identity	/1
Asks an open question to begin the consultation	/1
Enquires about symptoms of pain and prolapse	/2
Enquires about associated symptoms such as: • urinary symptoms: frequency, urgency, dysuria, incontinence, recurrent urinary tract infections • bowel symptoms: change in bowel habit, obstructed defecation • discomfort or lack of sensation during sexual intercourse • genital skin changes, itching or soreness	/3
Enquires about aggravating risk factors for prolapse: • chronic cough • constipation	/2
Enquires about course of pain (improving, worsening or fluctuating) and whether intermittent or constant	/1
Establishes effect on life	/1
Takes a gynaecological history: • Date of last menstrual period • Duration and frequency of periods • Abnormal vaginal bleeding • Age at menarche and menopause • Menopausal symptoms: hot flushes, vaginal dryness • Cervical screening history: last checked, results, any treatment required • STI history: last checked, results, any treatment required	/2
Takes an obstetric history: • Any previous or current pregnancies	/1

• Enquires about modes of delivery • Any miscarriages or terminations	
Takes a sexual history: • Enquires if sexually active and with whom • Sensitively enquires about consent • Establishes whether regular or casual partner • Use of contraception • Enquires about partner's STI history	**/1**
Enquires about past medical and surgical history	**/1**
Enquires about drug history and allergies	**/1**
Enquires about family history	**/1**
Enquires about social history • Student or employment status • Living arrangements • Smoking, alcohol and use of recreational drugs	**/1**
Gains patient's ideas, concerns and expectations	**/1**
Chunks and checks	**/1**
Provides a leaflet	**/1**
Appropriately closes the consultation and thanks the patient	/1
Behaves in a professional manner	/1
Explains to the examiner what the most likely diagnosis is: • Pelvic organ prolapse	/1
Explains to the examiner what the next steps are • Examination: BMI, abdominal, bimanual and speculum (Sim's) including assessment of pelvic muscle tone • Management: conservative (pelvic floor exercises), medical (vaginal pessaries, topical oestrogen), or surgical • Refer to gynaecology	/4
Total	/30

Additional Information

Definition: Bulging of pelvic organs into the vagina due to a weakened pelvic floor.

- anterior prolapse: bladder bulges into the front wall (cystocele)
- posterior prolapse: rectum bulges into the back wall (rectocele)
- uterine prolapse: 3rd degree prolapse or procidentia
- vault prolapse: top of the vagina bulges down (common following hysterectomy)

Risk Factors

- pregnancy
- assisted delivery
- prolonged labour
- hysterectomy
- increasing age
- high BMI
- constipation
- persistent coughing
- heavy lifting
- joint hypermobility syndrome
- Ehlers-Danlos syndrome
- Marfan syndrome

Patients may be asymptomatic and the prolapse may only be noted on clinical examination.

Alternatively, patients may experience

- heaviness or dragging sensation
- backache
- urinary frequency, incontinence and recurrent urinary tract infections
- symptoms of outflow obstruction (urinary hesitancy, poor stream and incomplete emptying)
- Obstructed defecation (sometimes having to manually replace the prolapse to allow defection)
- discomfort or lack of sensation during sexual intercourse

Patients may also feel or be able to see the prolapse themselves.

Examination

- BMI
- Abdominal
- vaginal
- Sim's speculum

Management

- conservative
  - weight loss
  - manage chronic cough e.g. stop smoking
  - prevent or treat constipation e.g. dietary changes, laxatives
  - avoid heavy lifting
  - avoid strenuous exercise
  - pelvic floor exercises for at least 16 weeks
- medical
  - topical oestrogen
  - vaginal pessary
    - will require follow up every 6 months
- surgical
  - vaginal hysterectomy +/- vaginal sacrospinous fixation with sutures
  - vaginal sacrospinous hysteropexy with sutures
  - manchester repair
  - sacro-hysteropexy with mesh
  - colpocleisis
  - for anterior prolapse
    - anterior repair without mesh
  - for posterior prolapse
    - posterior repair without mesh
  - for vault prolapse
    - vaginal sacrospinous fixation with sutures
    - sacrocolpopexy with mesh

Vaginal and speculum examination

Vignette

You are a junior doctor working in a GP practice. You have been asked to perform a vaginal and speculum examination on Miss Price, a 28-year-old lady, who has come in with post coital bleeding.

You do NOT have to take a history. You have 8 minutes for this station. At the end of your examination, summarise your findings to the examiner.

Patient brief

You are Sylvia Price, a 28-year-old lady who has presented to her GP due to postcoital bleeding. The candidate will demonstrate a vaginal and speculum examination.

Mark scheme

Introduces themselves, and confirms patients name and date of birth	/1
Washes hands and puts on gloves	/1
Explains the procedure to the patient and gains consent. Advise that the patient can request stop the examination at any time	/1
Asks if the patient is in any pain or if there if any chance the patient might be pregnant	/1
Offers the patient the chance to pass urine prior to the examination	/1
Offers a chaperone	/1
Comments on a general 'end of the bed' appearance	/1
Performs an abdominal examination, inspecting (1) and palpating (1) the abdomen for masses, tenderness and for inguinal lymphadenopathy	/2
Asks the patient to remove their underwear and position themselves in the modified lithotomy position ('bring your heels towards your bottom and then let your knees fall to the side'). Give them the privacy to do so	/1
Inspects and comments on the vulva (lesions, ulcers, visible discharge, bleeding, scars, cysts, whitening, erythema)	/2
Asks the patient to cough, inspecting for vaginal prolapse	/1
Warns the patient they are going to perform an internal exam	/1
Applied lubricant on gloved finger and parts the labia (using thumb and index finger) and inserts the index and middle fingers	/1
Palpates the vaginal walls and fornices for any irregularities or masses	/1
Bimanually palpates the uterus	/1
Bimanually palpates the adnexa	/1
Removes their fingers and comments on any blood/discharge on the glove	/1
Lubricates the speculum and warns patient they are about to insert it	/1
Parts the labia	/1

Gently inserts the speculum sideways, and once inserted, rotates the speculum back to 90 degrees	/1
Opens the speculum blades until a view of the cervix is obtained, and tightens the locking nut	/1
Comments on the appearance of the cervix (cervical os being open/closed, erosions around the os, cervical masses, ulceration, abnormal discharge/bleeding, polyps)	/2
Loosens the locking nut, partially closes the blades, and removes the speculum at 90 degrees, visualising the vaginal wall and it is removed	/1
Thanks the patient and allows them the chance to get dressed	/1
Disposes of gloves and washes hands	/1
Summarises findings to examiner	/1
Offers further examinations/investigations (vagina swabs, urinalysis, ultrasound)	/1
Total	/30

Additional information

There are several clinical findings at each stage of a vaginal and speculum examination:

Abdominal examination

Whilst you may not perform a full abdominal examination, it is important to inspect the abdomen, and observations such as scars, body habitus, and abdominal distension may aid your diagnosis.

On palpation of the abdomen, you may feel palpable masses, which you can further focus on during an internal examination. You may also feel tenderness – this can point to a gynaecological pathology, such as pelvic inflammatory disease, ovarian cysts, ectopic pregnancies etc, but it may also raise the possibility of surgical causes of abdominal pain such as appendicitis.

End of the bed

This is always an important part of any examination, particularly as it gives you a good idea of how unwell the patient is! You can also look out for secondary sexual characteristics.

Vulval inspection

Lesions could include many pathologies, but you want to rule out cancer

Ulcers are usually suggestive of genital herpes and are usually very painful!

Discharge can be normal, but can be suggestive of chlamydia/ gonorrhoea/ trichomoniasis (may be cloudy or pus like), candida ('cottage cheese'), or bacterial vaginosis (watery and 'fish' smelling)

Bleeding could be normal if the patient is menstruating, but may suggest fibroids, polyps, ectropion, infection, or malignancy

Scars would usually suggest previous surgery, but may also be present in lichen sclerosis

Cysts may occur when Bartholin's glands get blocked or infected.

Whitening may occur with lichen sclerosis. This is an inflammatory condition causing white thickened patches, which are very itchy and can cause scarring. It has a risk for malignant transformation

Erythema may occur in a variety of infective and inflammatory processes

Prolapse can be identified if a visible bulge protrudes from the vagina. It can be exacerbating by coughing and so asking the patient to cough forms a useful part of the examination

Internal Examination

Vaginal walls: a palpable mass in the vaginal wall may just be a cyst or fibroid, but it is important to rule out malignancy. The fornices are felt further up in the vagina and around the sides of the cervix. Again, you are feeling for a palpable mass

Cervix: move your fingers over the cervix to feel for whether it is smooth or irregular (irregular may suggest malignancy), and for in there is cervical excitation (suggestive of PID or ectopic pregnancy). Cervical cancer may also be very tender on examination

Uterus: to examine the uterus, you use your dominant hand to push upwards from the cervix, whilst using your other hand to simultaneously palpate the fundus (lower abdomen).

In a normal female, a palpable uterus is about the size of her fist. It may be larger with fibroids, pregnancy, or malignancy. You can also comment on if the uterus in anteverted or retroverted, and comment on any characteristics of the surface.

A similar technique should be used to palpate the fornices laterally, whilst palpating the left and right iliac fossa, feeling for any masses around the ovaries

Speculum examination

This primarily aids visualisation of the cervix. Erosions can suggest ectropion, but also malignancy. Ulceration can occur with genital herpes. Abnormal discharge may also be suggestive of an infective process. However, the main thing to rule out with cervical abnormalities, is CIN or cervical cancer.

Vaginal Discharge

Vignette

You are a final year medical student on your placement at a sexual health clinic and you have been asked to see Jenny Wong, a 17-year-old student who has come in with a change in vaginal discharge.

Please take a history. The examiner will stop you at 7 minutes to ask you a few questions.

Patient Brief

Presenting Complaint:

You introduce yourself (Jenny Wong, 5/5/03) and explain that you have noticed a change in your vaginal discharge. You are embarrassed to talk about it but with sensitive questioning, you explain that you have had thinner, whiter, and fishy smelling discharge for the past two weeks.

History of Presenting Complaint:

You do not have any genital itching or soreness, and you have not noticed any abnormal vaginal bleeding. You do not have any abdominal or pelvic pain. You do not have any urinary nor systemic symptoms. You have never had this symptom before so you cannot tell if it is related to your menstrual cycle. You have not tried any treatments yet and you do not use any feminine hygiene products.

Obstetric and Gynaecological History:

Your last menstrual period was 3 weeks ago. They usually last 5 to 7 days and you have a regular 28-day cycle. You do not have any abnormal vaginal bleeding. You are not having cervical screening and you have never been tested for STIs. You have never been pregnant.

Sexual History:

You have a boyfriend of 6 months and you had sex for the first time 2 months ago. You have had oral sex more recently. These encounters have all been consensual and you normally use condoms. He is the same age as you and he is English. You do not know if he has ever been checked for STIs, but he says he has never had sex before your relationship.

Past Medical and Surgical History:

You do not have any medical conditions and you have not had any operations.

Drug History and Allergies:

You do not take any regular medication and you do not have any allergies that you know of.

Family History:

You have no family history of any conditions.

Social History:

You are a college student living with your parents. You do not smoke and occasionally drink at parties. You have never tried recreational drugs.

Ideas, Concerns and Expectations:
You are not sure what is causing this change in vaginal discharge, but you are embarrassed and do not know what to do.

The examiner will now ask the candidate some questions.

3) What examination and investigations should be offered?
4) What is the most likely diagnosis and management?
5) How is the diagnosis of Bacterial Vaginosis made?

Mark Scheme

Introduces self with full name and role	/1
Confirms patient's identity	/1
Asks an open question to begin the consultation	/1
Enquires about the characteristics of the discharge • Onset and duration • Colour, odour, and consistency	/2
Enquires about associated symptoms such as: • Genital skin changes, itching or soreness • Abnormal vaginal bleeding: post-coital, intermenstrual, menorrhagia, dysmenorrhoea • Abdominal or pelvic pain • Dysuria • General malaise, fever, weight loss, rashes or joint swellings	/2
Enquires about previous episodes • Relation to menstrual cycle	/1
Enquires about relieving or exacerbating factors • Prescription or over the counter treatments • Use of vaginal products such as douches, deodorants, or washes	/1
Enquires about effect on life	/1
Takes a gynaecological history: • Date of last menstrual period • Duration and frequency of periods • Abnormal vaginal bleeding • Cervical screening history: last checked, results, any treatment required • STI history: last checked, results, any treatment required	/2
Takes an obstetric history: • Any previous or current pregnancies • Any miscarriages or terminations	/1
Takes a sexual history: • Most recent sexual encounter • Sensitively enquires about consent • Establishes whether regular or casual partner	/2

• Enquires about sex and nationality of partner • Enquires about type of sex • Use of contraception • Enquires about partner's STI history • Enquires about any other partners in last 3 months in the same manner	
Enquires about past medical and surgical history	/1
Enquires about drug history and allergies	/1
Enquires about family history	/1
Enquires about social history • Occupation and housing • Smoking, alcohol and use of recreational drugs	/1
Gains patient's ideas, concerns, and expectations	/1
Provides a leaflet	/1
Appropriately closes the consultation and thanks the patient	/1
Behaves in a professional manner	/1
Explains to the examiner what examinations and investigations should be offered • Systemic, abdominal, bimanual and speculum examinations • High or low vaginal swab for Gram staining, NAATs and culture • Testing for HIV, syphilis, and hepatitis if strong sexual health risk factors	/3
Explains to the examiner what the most likely diagnosis is and its management • Bacterial vaginosis • 400mg oral metronidazole to be taken twice daily for 5 to 7 days	/2
How is the diagnosis of Bacterial vaginosis made? • Amsel's criteria: • Thin, white, yellow, homogeneous discharge • Clue cells on microscopy • pH of vaginal fluid >4.5 • Release of a fishy odour on adding alkali—10% potassium hydroxide (KOH) solution.	/2

At least three of the four criteria should be present for a confirmed diagnosis.	
Total	/30

Additional Information

Normal physiological discharge is usually white or clear with no offensive smell.
It can vary during menstruation, ovulation, sexual arousal, pregnancy and with use of contraception. It usually decreases around menopause due to lower oestrogen levels.

Abnormal vaginal discharge usually has a change of colour, consistency, volume, or odour.
It may be associated with genital itching, soreness, dysuria, pelvic or abdominal pain, or abnormal vaginal bleeding.

Infective causes

Bacterial vaginosis (most common)

- caused by an overgrowth of anaerobic bacteria especially *Gardnerella vaginalis*
- presents with a fishy-smelling, thin, grey, or white homogenous discharge
- usually not associated with genital itching or soreness
- investigate with high or low vaginal swabs for Gram staining
    - pH of vaginal discharge should be more than 4.5
- treat with 400mg oral metronidazole to be taken twice daily for 5 to 7 days
    - or a single 2g dose of oral metronidazole
    - or topical 0.75% metronidazole for 5 days
    - or topical 2% clindamycin for 7 days
- treatment not required if asymptomatic and not pregnant or undergone a termination of pregnancy
- test of cure not required

Vaginal candidiasis

- caused by the fungus *Candida albicans*
- presents with a white, odourless, and curd-like discharge
- associated with vulval itching and superficial soreness
- may have erythema, fissuring, oedema, and excoriation on examination
- investigation usually not required
    - pH of vaginal discharge should be less than 4.5
    - treat with topical clotrimazole or pessary of oral fluconazole or itraconazole
- test of cure not required

Trichomoniasis

- sexually transmitted infection caused by the protozoa *Trichomonas vaginalis*
- presents with fishy-smelling, yellow or green frothy discharge
- associated with vulval itching and soreness, and dysuria
- may have cervicitis ("strawberry cervix") on speculum examination
- investigate with high or low vaginal swabs for Gram staining
    - pH of vaginal discharge should be more than 4.5
- should refer to Genito-urinary medicine
- treat with 400mg oral metronidazole to be taken twice daily for 5 to 7 days
    - or a single 2g dose of oral metronidazole
- treat current partner and any sexual contacts within the last 4 weeks
    - offer full STI screening to patient and sexual contacts
- should be followed up regarding symptoms, contract tracing and STI screening results
- advise abstinence until 1 week after treatment and follow up are complete
- test of cure not required

Endocervical *Chlamydia trachomatis*

- may cause localised cervicitis or ascending pelvic inflammatory disease
- may present with abnormal vaginal discharge, post-coital or intermenstrual bleeding, dysuria, deep dyspareunia, or lower abdominal pain
- investigate with endocervical or vulvovaginal swabs, or 1st catch urine for NAATs
- should refer to Genito-urinary medicine
- treat with 100mg oral doxycycline to be taken twice daily for 7 days (1st line)
    - treat current partner
- offer full STI screening to patient and current partner
- advise abstinence until treatment is complete
- offer repeat testing to those under 25 years old 3 to 6 months after treatment

Endocervical *Neisseria gonorrhoeae*

- may cause localised cervicitis or ascending pelvic inflammatory disease

- may present with abnormal vaginal discharge, post-coital or intermenstrual bleeding, dysuria, deep dyspareunia, or lower abdominal pain
- investigate with vulvovaginal swab for NAATs and culture
- should refer to Genito-urinary medicine
- treat with a single 1g dose of intramuscular ceftriaxone (1st line)
    - or a single 500mg dose of oral ciprofloxacin (if sensitivities are known)
- offer full STI screening to patient and any sexual contacts within the last 3 months
- advise abstinence until treatment in complete
- should be followed up in 1 week with test of cure

<u>Non-infective causes</u>

- Retained foreign body such as tampon, condom, or vaginal sponge
- Inflammation secondary to allergy or irritation due to deodorants, lubricants, or disinfectants
- Vulval, vaginal, cervical, or endometrial tumours
- Atrophic vaginitis if post-menopausal
- Cervical ectopy or polyps
- Fistulae
- Recent childbirth (with perineal or vaginal lacerations, or episiotomy)
- Recent vaginal surgery

Abbreviations

ABG: Arterial blood gas

ACE-i: Angiotensin converting enzyme inhibitors

ALP: Alkaline Phosphatase

ALT: Alanine Aminotransferase

AST: Aspartate Aminotransferase

AVPU scale: "Alert, verbal, pain, unresponsive" scale

B-HCG: Beta human chorionic gonadotrophin

BMI: Body Mass Index

BD: Twice daily

BP: Blood pressure

CBG: Capillary blood glucose

CBT: Cognitive behavioural therapy

CIN: Cervical intraepithelial neoplasia

CMV: Cytomegalovirus

COCP: Combined oral contraceptive pill

CRP: C-reactive protein

CSF: Cerebrospinal fluid

CTG: Cardiotocography

CTPA: CT pulmonary angiography

DCDA: Dichorionic diamniotic (twins)

DVT: Deep vein thrombosis

EBV: Epstein-Barr virus

ECG: Electrocardiogram

ECT: Electroconvulsive therapy

ECV: External cephalic version

FBC: Full blood count

FFP: Fresh frozen plasma

FSH: follicle stimulating hormone

FSRH: Faculty of Sexual & Reproductive Healthcare

GCS: Glasgow Coma Scale

GnRH: gonadotropin releasing hormone

GP: General practice

GTD: Gestational trophoblastic disease

HbA1C: Glycated haemoglobin

HELLP: Haemolysis, elevated liver enzymes, low platelets

HIV: Human immunodeficiency virus

HPV: Human pappilomavirus

HR: Heart rate

IM: Intramuscular

IUD: Intrauterine device

IUGR: Intrauterine growth restriction

IV: Intravenous

IVF: In vitro fertilisation

JVP: Jugular venous pressure

L: Litre

LARC: Long acting reversible contraception

LH: luteinising hormone

LLETZ: Large loop excision of the transformation zone

LMP: Last menstrual period

LFTs: Liver function tests

MCDA: Monochorionic diamniotic (twins)

MCMA: Monochorionic monoamniotic (twins)

NAATs: Nucleic acid amplification tests

NHS: National health service

NICE: National institute for health and care excellence

OD: Once daily

PCOS: Polycystic ovarian syndrome

PE: Pulmonary embolism

PID: Pelvic inflammatory disease

PIH: Pregnancy induced hypertension

PND: Postnatal depression

POP: Progesterone only pill

PPH: Postpartum haemorrhage

PROM: Prelabour rupture of membranes

PPROM: Preterm prelabour rupture of membranes

QDS: Four times daily

qSOFA: quick Sepsis Related Organ Failure Assessment

RA: Room air

RBC: Red blood cells

RR: Respiratory rate

RUQ: Right upper quadrant

SaO2: Oxygen saturations

STI: Sexually transmitted infection

T: Temperature

TB: Tuberculosis

TDS: Three times daily

TFTs: Thyroid function tests

TOP: Termination of pregnancy

TORCH: Toxoplasmosis, Other agents, Rubella, Cytomegalovirus and Herpes simplex

TTTS: Twin to twin transfusion syndrome

TVT: Tension Free vaginal tape

U&Es: Urea and electrolytes

UK MEC: UK medical eligibility criteria (contraception)

UPSI: Unprotected Sexual Intercourse

US: Ultrasound

UTI: Urinary tract infection

VBG: Venous blood gas

V/Q scan: Ventilation-perfusion scan

VTE: Venous thromboembolism

WHO: World Health Organisation

References

Antepartum Haemorrhage

1. The ABCDE Approach [Internet]. Resuscitation Council UK; 2015. Available from: https://www.resus.org.uk/library/2015-resuscitation-guidelines/abcde-approach#additional-information

2. Antepartum Haemorrhage (Green-top Guideline No. 63) [Internet]. 1st ed. London: Royal College of Obstetricians and Gynaecologists; 2011. Available from: https://www.rcog.org.uk/globalassets/documents/guidelines/gtg_63.pdf

Booking appointment

3. Antenatal care for uncomplicated pregnancies Clinical guideline [CG62] [internet] NICE. 2019. Available at: https://www.nice.org.uk/guidance/cg62

CTG Interpretation

4. CTG interpretation and further management | eLearning [Internet]. Elearning.rcog.org.uk. 2020. Available from: https://elearning.rcog.org.uk/obstetrics/electronic-fetal-monitoring/ctg-interpretation-and-further

5. Interpretation of cardiotocograph traces [Internet]. National Institute for Health and Care Excellence; 2017. Available from: https://www.nice.org.uk/guidance/cg190/resources/interpretation-of-cardiotocograph-traces-pdf-248732173

Ectopic Pregnancy

6.Elson CJ, et al on behalf of the Royal College of Obstetricians and Gynaecologists. Diagnosis and management of ectopic pregnancy. BJOG 2016;.123:e15–e55

Gestational Diabetes Mellitus

7. Diabetes In Pregnancy: Management From Preconception To The Postnatal Period [internet] NICE. 2015 Available at: <https://www.nice.org.uk/Guidance/NG3> [Accessed 17 October 2020].

8. Caughey, A., 2020. Gestational diabetes mellitus: Obstetric issues and management. [internet] Uptodate.com. Available at: <https://www.uptodate.com/contents/gestational-diabetes-mellitus-obstetric-issues-and-management[accessed 17 October 2020].

Hyperemesis Gravidarum

9. The Management of Nausea and Vomiting of Pregnancy and Hyperemesis Gravidarum (Green-top Guideline No. 69) [Internet]. 1st ed. London: Royal College of Obstetricians and Gynaecologists; 2016. Available from: https://www.rcog.org.uk/globalassets/documents/guidelines/green-top-guidelines/gtg69-hyperemesis.pdf

10. The Management of Gestational Trophoblastic Disease (Green-top Guideline No. 38) [Internet]. 1st ed. London: Royal College of Obstetricians and Gynaecologists; 2010. Available from: https://www.rcog.org.uk/globalassets/documents/guidelines/gtg_38.pdf

11. Dean C, Shemar M, Ostrowski G, Painter R. Management of severe pregnancy sickness and hyperemesis gravidarum. BMJ. 2018;(363):k5000.

Hypertension in Pregnancy

12. Recommendations | Hypertension in pregnancy: diagnosis and management | Guidance | NICE [Internet]. Nice.org.uk. 2020 [cited 21 September 2020]. Available from: https://www.nice.org.uk/guidance/ng133/chapter/Recommendations

13. Burton G, Redman C, Roberts J, Moffett A. Pre-eclampsia: pathophysiology and clinical implications. BMJ. 2019;(366):l2381.

Labour

14. The mechanism of normal labour and birth | eLearning [Internet]. Elearning.rcog.org.uk. 2019 [cited 21 September 2020]. Available from: https://elearning.rcog.org.uk//mechanisms-normal-labour-and-birth/mechanism-normal-labour-and-birth

15. Overview | Inducing labour | Guidance | NICE [Internet]. Nice.org.uk. 2008 [cited 21 September 2020]. Available from: https://www.nice.org.uk/guidance/cg70

16. Overview | Intrapartum care for healthy women and babies | Guidance | NICE [Internet]. Nice.org.uk. 2014 [cited 21 September 2020]. Available from: https://www.nice.org.uk/guidance/cg190

Miscarriage

17. Ectopic pregnancy and miscarriage: diagnosis and initial management NICE guideline [NG126].[internet] Nice.org.uk. 2019 . Available from: https://www.nice.org.uk/guidance/ng126

18. Prager, S. Pregnancy loss (miscarriage): Risk factors, etiology, clinical manifestations, and diagnostic evaluation [internet] UpToDate. 2020.

Available from: https://www.uptodate.com/contents/pregnancy-loss-miscarriage-risk-factors-etiology-clinical-manifestations-and-diagnostic-evaluation#H1971624904

Obstetric Cholestasis

19.Itch in pregnancy [internet] NICE CKS. 2020. [Accessed 17/10/2020] Available at: https://cks.nice.org.uk/topics/itch-in-pregnancy/

20.Obstetric Cholestasis, Green –top Guideline No. 43. [internet] RCOG. 2011. [Accessed 17/10/2020] Available at: https://www.rcog.org.uk/globalassets/documents/guidelines/gtg_43.pdf

Postnatal Check-up

21. Postnatal care up to 8 weeks after birth. Clinical guideline [CG37] [internet] NICE. Available at :https://www.nice.org.uk/guidance/cg37

22. Jakes, A. et al The maternal six week postnatal check. *BMJ 2019;367:l6482*

Postnatal Depression

23. Management of Women with Mental Health Issues during Pregnancy and the Postnatal Period [Internet]. Rcog.org.uk. 2011. Available from: https://www.rcog.org.uk/globalassets/documents/guidelines/managementwomenmentalhealthgoodpractice14.pdf

24. SIGN 127 • Management of perinatal mood disorders [Internet]. Sign.ac.uk. 2012. Available from: https://www.sign.ac.uk/assets/sign127_update.pdf

25. Overview | Antenatal and postnatal mental health: clinical management and service guidance | Guidance | NICE [Internet]. Nice.org.uk. 2014. Available from: https://www.nice.org.uk/guidance/cg192

Postpartum Pyrexia

26. Bacterial Sepsis following Pregnancy (Green-top Guideline No. 64b) [Internet]. London: Royal College of Obstetricians and Gynaecologists; 2012. Available from: https://www.rcog.org.uk/globalassets/documents/guidelines/gtg_64b.pdf

27. Sepsis: Risk stratification tools [Internet]. National Institute for Health and Care Excellence; 2017. Available from: https://www.nice.org.uk/guidance/ng51/resources/algorithm-for-managing-suspected-sepsis-in-adults-and-young-people-aged-18-years-and-over-in-an-acute-hospital-setting-2551485715

28. qSOFA :: quick Sepsis Related Organ Failure Assessment [Internet]. Qsofa.org. 2020. Available from: https://qsofa.org/

29. Thromboembolic Disease in Pregnancy and the Puerperium: Acute Management (Green-top Guideline No. 37b) [Internet]. London: Royal College of Obstetricians and Gynaecologists; 2015. Available from: https://www.rcog.org.uk/globalassets/documents/guidelines/gtg-37b.pdf

Postpartum Haemorrhage

30.The ABCDE Approach [Internet]. Resuscitation Council UK; 2015. Available from: https://www.resus.org.uk/library/2015-resuscitation-guidelines/abcde-approach#additional-information

31.Prevention and Management of Postpartum Haemorrhage (Green-top Guideline No. 52) [Internet]. London: Royal College of Obstetricians and Gynaecologists; 2016. Available from: https://obgyn.onlinelibrary.wiley.com/doi/epdf/10.1111/1471-0528.14178

32.Updated WHO Recommendation on Tranexamic Acid for the Treatment of Postpartum Haemorrhage [Internet]. World Health Organisation; 2017. Available from: https://apps.who.int/iris/bitstream/handle/10665/259379/WHO-RHR-17.21-eng.pdf?sequence=1

Twin pregnancy

33. Overview | Twin and triplet pregnancy | Guidance | NICE [Internet]. Nice.org.uk. 2019. Available from: https://www.nice.org.uk/guidance/ng137

34. Pregnant with twins [Internet]. nhs.uk. 2019. Available from: https://www.nhs.uk/conditions/pregnancy-and-baby/what-causes-twins/

Cervical Smear

35. Obtaining Valid Consent [Internet]. Rcog.org.uk. 2015. Available from: https://www.rcog.org.uk/globalassets/documents/guidelines/clinical-governance-advice/cga6.pdf

36. Cervical screening: leaflet for women considering screening [Internet]. GOV.UK. 2012. Available from: https://www.gov.uk/government/publications/cervical-screening-description-in-brief

Contraception Counselling

37. Contraception - NICE Pathways [Internet]. Pathways.nice.org.uk. 2020. Available from: https://pathways.nice.org.uk/pathways/contraception

38. UKMEC April 2016 (Amended September 2019) - Faculty of Sexual and Reproductive Healthcare [Internet]. Fsrh.org. 2019. Available from: https://www.fsrh.org/standards-and-guidance/documents/ukmec-2016/

39. Combined pill [Internet]. nhs.uk. 2020. Available from: https://www.nhs.uk/conditions/contraception/combined-contraceptive-pill/

Dyspareunia

40. BASHH Guidelines [Internet]. Bashhguidelines.org. 2019. Available from: https://www.bashhguidelines.org/current-guidelines/systemic-presentation-and-complications/pid-2019/

41. Pelvic inflammatory disease [Internet]. National Institute for Health and Care Excellence. 2019. Available from: https://cks.nice.org.uk/topics/pelvic-inflammatory-disease/#!scenario

42. Acute pelvic inflammatory disease [Internet]. London: Royal College of Obstetricians and Gynaecologists; 2016. Available from: https://www.rcog.org.uk/globalassets/documents/patients/patient-information-leaflets/gynaecology/pi-acute-pid.pdf

Emergency Contraception

43. Contraception - emergency [Internet]. National Institute for Health and Care Excellence. 2020. Available from: https://cks.nice.org.uk/topics/contraception-emergency/#!management

44. FSRH Guideline: Emergency Contraception [Internet]. The Faculty of Sexual & Reproductive Healthcare; 2017. Available from: https://www.fsrh.org/standards-and-guidance/documents/ceu-clinical-guidance-emergency-contraception-march-2017/

Endometriosis

45.Endometriosis: diagnosis and management. NICE guideline [NG73] [internet] NICE. 2017. Available at: https://www.nice.org.uk/guidance/ng73

46.Schenken, R. Endometriosis.: Treatment of pelvic pain. [internet] UpToDate Available at: ttps://www.uptodate.com/contents/endometriosis-treatment-of-pelvic-pain

Irregular menstrual bleeding

47. Polycystic Ovary Syndrome, Long-term Consequences (Green-top Guideline No. 33) [Internet]. Royal College of Obstetricians and Gynaecologists. 2014. Available from: https://www.rcog.org.uk/en/guidelines-research-services/guidelines/gtg33/

48. Scenario. Secondary amenorrhoea | Management | Amenorrhoea | CKS | NICE [Internet]. Cks.nice.org.uk. 2019. Available from: https://cks.nice.org.uk/topics/amenorrhoea/management/secondary-amenorrhoea/

Menorrhagia

49. Heavy menstrual bleeding. NICE guideline [NG88] [internet] NICE, 2020. Available at: https://www.nice.org.uk/guidance/ng88

50. Fraser, IS et al. Abnormal uterine bleeding in reproductive age women: Terminology and PALM-COEIN etiology classification [internet] UpToDate. 2019. Available at: https://www.uptodate.com/contents/abnormal-uterine-bleeding-in-reproductive-age-women-terminology-and-palm-coein-etiology-classification

51. Munro, M. et al FIGO classification system (PALM-COEIN) for causes of abnormal uterine bleeding in nongravid women of reproductive age. International Journal of Gynecology & Obstetrics. 2011;113(1);3-13

Ovarian Torsion

52. Damigos, E et al. An update on the diagnosis and management of ovarian torsion. The obstetrician & Gynaecologist 2012;12:229-36

53. Skandhan. A, and Dixon. A et al. Ovarian torsion [internet] Radiopaedia. [Accessed 13/07/20] Available at: https://radiopaedia.org/articles/ovarian-torsion?lang=gb

54. Ovarian torsion. [internet] BMJ Best practice. Available at: https://bestpractice.bmj.com/topics/en-gb/792

55. Laufer, M. Ovarian and fallopian tube torsion [internet] UpToDate (2020) Available at: https://www.uptodate.com/contents/ovarian-and-fallopian-tube-torsion

Overactive Bladder Syndrome

56. Lukacz, E. Evaluation of females with urinary incontinence [internet] UpToDate. 2020. Available from: https://www.uptodate.com/contents/evaluation-of-females-with-urinary-incontinence

57. Urinary incontinence and pelvic organ prolapse in women: management. NICE guideline [NG123] [internet] NICE. 2019. Available from https://www.nice.org.uk/guidance/ng123/

Postmenopausal Bleeding

58. Postmenopausal bleeding [Internet]. NHS. 2020. Available from: https://www.nhs.uk/conditions/post-menopausal-bleeding/#:~:text=There%20can%20be%20several%20causes,that%20are%20usually%20non%2Dcancerous

59. Brand A. The woman with postmenopausal bleeding. Australian Family Physician [Internet]. 2007;36(3):1-5. Available from: https://www.racgp.org.au/afpbackissues/2007/200703/200703brand.pdf

60. Suspected cancer: recognition and referral [Internet]. National Institute for Health and Care Excellence; 2015. Available from: https://www.nice.org.uk/guidance/ng12/resources/suspected-cancer-recognition-and-referral-pdf-1837268071621

Termination of Pregnancy

61. Overview | Abortion care | Guidance | NICE [Internet]. Nice.org.uk. 2019. Available from: https://www.nice.org.uk/guidance/NG140

62. The Care of Women Requesting Induced Abortion [Internet]. Rcog.org.uk. 2011. Available from: https://www.rcog.org.uk/globalassets/documents/guidelines/abortion-guideline_web_1.pdf

63. Britain's Abortion Law | Briefings | Advocacy | BPAS [Internet]. Bpas.org. 2020. Available from: https://www.bpas.org/get-involved/campaigns/briefings/abortion-law/

Uterine Prolapse

64. Pelvic organ prolapse [Internet]. NHS. 2020. Available from: https://www.nhs.uk/conditions/pelvic-organ-prolapse/

65. Pelvic organ prolapse [Internet]. London: Royal College of Obstetricians and Gynaecologists; 2013. Available from: https://www.rcog.org.uk/globalassets/documents/patients/patient-information-leaflets/gynaecology/pi-pelvic-organ-prolapse.pdf

66. Urinary incontinence and pelvic organ prolapse in women: management [Internet]. National Institute for Health and Care Excellence; 2019. Available from: https://www.nice.org.uk/guidance/ng123/resources/urinary-incontinence-and-pelvic-organ-prolapse-in-women-management-pdf-66141657205189

Vaginal and Speculum Examination

67. Gynaecological Examinations: Guidelines for Specialist Practice [Internet]. Elearning.rcog.org.uk. 2002. Available from:

https://elearning.rcog.org.uk/sites/default/files/Communication%20skills/rcog_gynaeexams4.pdf

68. Vaginal Examination (PV) - OSCE Guide | Geeky Medics [Internet]. Geeky Medics. 2020. Available from: https://geekymedics.com/bimanual-vaginal-examination/

69. Speculum Examination - OSCE Guide | Geeky Medics [Internet]. Geeky Medics. 2020. Available from: https://geekymedics.com/speculum-examination-osce-guide/

Vaginal Discharge

70. Vaginal discharge [Internet]. National Institute for Health and Care Excellence. 2019. Available from: https://cks.nice.org.uk/topics/vaginal-discharge/#!topicSummary

www.ingramcontent.com/pod-product-compliance
Ingram Content Group UK Ltd.
Pitfield, Milton Keynes, MK11 3LW, UK
UKHW022025190726
13853UKWH00005B/2117